1988

YOGA AND PRAYER

There are innumerable experts on yoga, and many demand no more from the discipline than relaxation and health. But here is one who shows how yoga is able to lead to a close union with God, and a more creative approach to prayer. The author was born into an atheist family, and began to practice yoga purely for health and self-discipline. When she was converted to Christianity she believed at first that yoga would be superfluous, but a meeting in 1956 with Jean Déchanet (the author of *Christian Yoga*, *Ten Lessons in Yoga* and *Yoga and God*) showed her how to relate yoga disciplines and Christian spirituality, and that hatha yoga was both an effective natural discipline and one that makes the practitioner more available to God and more aware of his compassion.

This eminently practical book is the fruit of that discovery, and of solitary and group practice and research. It will help those who, by means of hatha yoga exercises, wish to put their bodies in tune with the infinite. The book contains a wealth of tips on relaxation, correct body posture, prayerful attitudes and exercises, and recipes for a healthy diet. Numerous diagrams illustrate the variety of recommended postures and movements.

In the same series:

TEN LESSONS IN YOGA J.-M. Déchanet

CHRISTIAN YOGA J.-M. Déchanet

YOGA AND GOD J.-M. Déchanet

YOGA FOR CHILDREN Martina Luchs

THE GRACE OF ZEN Karlfried Dürckheim *et al.*

THE PRACTICE OF MEDITATION Klemens Tilmann

MEDITATION IN DEPTH Klemens Tilmann

MEDITATION AND YOU Klemens Tilmann

AS THE BIRDS DO: PARABLES OF LONELINESS J. Drake-Brockman

YOGA AND PRAYER

Michaëlle

Search Press · London
Christian Classics · Westminster, Maryland

First published in Great Britain, associated territories, and Ireland
in 1980 by Search Press Limited, 2–10 Jerdan Place, London SW6 5PT
and in the USA by Christian Classics, Westminster, Maryland

First published in French in 1977 by Les Editions du Cerf,
29, bd Latour-Maubourg, Paris, France
Copyright © Les Editions du Cerf 1977
This translation and adaptation copyright © Search Press Ltd 1980
All rights reserved. No part of this publication may be reproduced in
any form or by any means without the previous written permission of
Search Press Limited.

Illustrated by a Poor Clare
Translated and adapted by Diana Cumming

ISBN 0 85532 437 6
ISBN (USA) 0-87061-059-7

Typeset by Input Typesetting Ltd, London
Printed in Great Britain by A. Wheaton & Co. Ltd.

CONTENTS

INTRODUCTION

Life is full of problems. Sooner or later, everyone has to cope with difficulties of one kind or another, but finding an effective way of overcoming them may well present the greatest difficulty of all. There is a great need for a tried and true method of facing the 'slings and arrows of outrageous fortune'. Yoga fulfils that need.

It has been proved again and again that yoga really works. This unique discipline is available to all, yet many deprive themselves of its extraordinary advantages. To experience life at a deeper level and thus become a whole person, a complete human being, is not the right of a favoured few, but of all humanity.

Hatha yoga is the music of the soul, and God is the source of life. This music flows into the soul, uplifting and inspiring it so that it is prepared for a union with God. Belief in yoga does not preclude belief in prayer, or *vice versa*; the state of prayer is a state of harmony with self, so that the whole being is in harmony with God. A calm mind produces a completely relaxed body, but disordered thoughts prevent absolute surrender. Not that this book tries to claim that yoga is essential to prayer; it is offered as an aid and a supplement.

This text is a testimony to endeavour, and to the fruits of that endeavour. Each personal experience is recounted with absolute veracity. This book is not a blue-print for correct methods of prayer; it is simply the sum of long experience.

Before embarking upon any major project, Jesus himself always retired to pray. Prayer is like a well full of God's love, always available for nourishment and refreshment. Mankind was created by love, so love alone can erase man's miseries. The divine hands tenderly created man in God's image – indelibly, eternally; come what may. This is how the history of love between God and his beloved children began, and such a beginning ensures that finally, no matter how degenerate a man may be, when the phenomenon of communication with God takes place he will change completely in thought, word, and deed. The generosity of God is unlimited; the human mind cannot even begin to comprehend the extent of his love and mercy. If man could only reject his prejudices and banish his doubts, he could completely open himself up and be ready to accept God, and achieve oneness with him. A unique personal contact with the divine presence is attainable during prayer only if the soul is willing and able to accept instruction, and this can be given only by living cells which are functioning correctly. These cells are constantly renewed by the soul itself. Prayer assists the soul in the process of calming the nerves and preventing the dissipation of mental energies, and so inner peace is achieved. The inner self must be contacted and brought to a state of relaxed concentration before it can both accept and make proper use of God's grace.

Man, operating as he does on the principle that the whole is the sum of each complementary part, is a perfect creation. But mankind makes the grave mistake of trying to dissociate elements which in theory may function very well independently, but in practice do nothing of the kind. They should always function in unison, but attention is seldom paid to the organisation of the different parts, so they are unable to operate as a unified team. In the cosmos, certain laws will eternally prevail; man, who is in partnership with the cosmos, was created one, and man is one – in mind, body and soul. The process of prayer restores man's harmonious ebb and flow. Just as day and night submit to the positive and negative influences of the sun and moon, so the two 'male' and 'female' forces exist equally in every individual, and balance themselves within the context of the cosmos. Man and his environment are complementary (for instance, a man and a tree). Every particle of the physical body of each individual is a point of resonance, and just as the resonance of music or any vibrations will produce a reaction, emotional resonance will affect the individual psyche. Changes of attitude and posture lead to a deeper level of prayer. This is quite logical, as each element of the body has been created with such precision that it relies upon the totality of the being. Such an apparently simple thing as the position of the hands – open or closed, palms upturned or down – will affect the quality of prayer. The first quality of prayer is sincerity, without which all other considerations are futile. The result of the following experiment will indicate the relation between prayer and posture:

First, clench the fists and tighten the jaw.

Relax.

Smile, open the hands, raise the arms loosely from the body, as though welcoming some much-loved person.

The vibrations will be felt in the soul.

I THE BODY AND SPIRITUALITY

1. RELAXATION AND AVAILABILITY TO GOD

A. He leads me to the still waters; He restoreth my soul (Ps. 22, 2)

It is always easier to draw nearer to God during a period of relaxation. Relaxation stops all aggravation and nervous movement. If you are relaxed you do not fidget, and you are at liberty to cultivate harmony in thought and gesture. This state will finally bring the peace described so accurately by the psalmist (Ps. 4 and 22). Then you can reach the full potential of all the complementary components of your being by means of beautiful and sacred gestures. These gestures spring from the depths of the inner self, and become powerful symbols.

The peace promised by God is attainable only by those who completely relinquish all problems (Hebrews 3 and 4). Access to this peace comes through surrender – unconditional surrender. This surrender to the divine tenderness must be without reserve. It should include the muscles, the nerves, the joints, the mind. This offering is a combination of every element of self, from the least to the greatest. Conceived by God, the master craftsman, the equipment available has been specially designed for this very purpose.

But there is a snag – our hectic life-style, with its constant interruptions and temptations. It does anything but predispose mankind to surrender. It results in either resistance or deterioration, neither of which states has anything in common with the conscious joy which procures the perfect peace promised in the Scriptures. Nevertheless, true values are sought universally, both by believers and non-believers. Even health authorities are beginning to recognize the need for some appropriate release from the constraints of modern life. Many schools of thought are trying to combat the problem by introducing various methods of relaxation and control, and most of them would be of benefit to everyone who is subjected to the anxieties of twentieth-century existence. The nerves of mankind are being worn to a frazzle, yet people are left to fend for

9

themselves. Even children are subjected to the most incredible hazards without being given the means of dealing with them. Most people are affected by frustrations, instead of living life as it should be lived.

It is particularly important for Christians to realize that relaxation can extend far beyond the limits of physical techniques; it can be transmuted into an experience of faith. This is the achievement of true communion between the child and the Father. It is that very approach to peace promised by God, which has an amazing effect upon the daily round and the common task.

Remember the following points:

– Decontraction exercises, which eliminate tension, may be practised during various activities.
– Maintaining the right attitude during other activities will supplement periods of relaxation devoted entirely to communion with God.
– The relaxation-surrender state may be achieved by prayer.

The exercise section includes instruction on progressive relaxation, as in cases of severe exhaustion or a lack of energy it is not advisable to try to cover the whole series all at once. The exercises should be increased gradually, with an occasional minutes rest. It is not a good idea to go on for too long without a break. Do not resist any drowsiness induced by the exercises. After all, relaxation is the object, so succumb! So much has been written on the subject of relaxation that a separation of the wheat from the chaff is necessary. Only the most valuable methods need be retained, but all relaxation instruction does have one point in common – simple muscular relaxation, using God-given natural means, is infinitely preferable to any hypnotic or quasi-hypnotic state. It is most inadvisable to try to relax by means of mental suggestion. Trances and hallucinations are products of the imagination; so are tensions and anxieties. The more demands which are made upon the imagination, the more will it be disturbed. The obvious answer to the problem is the use of the body. Here is first-rate equipment, at everyone's immediate disposal. Simple trial-and-error will show how it is best to be used. The body was made to function with a constant peak performance at every level. All that is needed is the right method.

The first clue to natural relaxation is the law of gravity. This suggests the necessity for a hard surface, so what could be more suitable than the ground, covered with some simple cloth. Here the muscles will be able to relax from all the pressures of modern life. Only those suffering from serious disabilities should use a soft surface, as under no circumstances should harm or discomfort be caused. A small cushion of folded cloth may be placed against the small of the back, and the spinal column, and under the thighs, as necessary. In order to keep the spine as flat as possible, keep your knees bent; the reasons for this will be given later. Wear very simple, loose attire. Girdles, belts, ties, spectacles, shoes,

10

stockings, and even jewellery are unsuitable. The removal of every unnecessary article of clothing or decoration is a step towards interior surrender. The rejection of all surplus trappings will liberate the bodily energies. The object is liberation and regeneration.

Relaxation is best achieved in a quiet, dimly-lit place, well-aired, but free from draughts and disturbances of any kind. Except for the relaxed position of a sleeping child (*Fig. 2*), it is essential that the body should be distributed evenly along the ground without curling up. No part of the body should be cramped, but it is best to move about gently, without trying to force the correct position; just fall into it naturally. Take care that the body is evenly distributed around the axis created by a line drawn from the bridge of the nose to the navel. The polarity between these two parts of the body, positive and negative, creates, conditions, and controls the very equilibrium which neutralises the mental processes. The malfunctioning of this equilibrium prevents surrender, impeding an awareness of the divine presence. Unfortunately, nowadays leisure provides little more relaxation than work. Both produce tensions and frustrations, so that self-renewal must be accomplished by other means.

Perpetual tensions produce mental reactions, and the results are distressing. They include fear, repression, and guilt. Even the effect of continuous noise is a confused inability to use sound judgment. It is difficult to dissociate the function of the 'body' from that of the brain, as they were originally intended to work in conjunction and produce a joint end-product. Any abuse of the body will have a bad effect on the mind; equally, a tormented mind will produce unfortunate physical effects. All these wretched states of mind and body cling like leeches. They uselessly absorb energy, injecting poisons into the bloodstream which interfere with the free circulation of energy. All this dissipation of energy is accentuated just when the batteries need recharging. Just as the engine is turned off when a car is parked, or the lights in a home switched off when the occupants retire, each individual should be sure to disconnect all the reactions of the body if a good night's rest is to be attained. If the responsibilities of the following day are to be fulfilled, the distribution of energy must take place during sleep, or sleep will not renew and refresh. During the night, there is a change in the polarity of the cosmos, the negativity of the moon being replaced by the positivity of the rising sun.

The body is subject to this transformation, and it is important that, during leisure hours, you should establish the correct equilibrium by the right kind of relaxation. The following methods of relaxation will help maintain the right balance.

1. Mechanical and muscular relaxation

Cats and dogs use this method constantly, and it is by far the most simple. A cat loves to lie fully stretched out lengthwise, either on her back or her stomach, while a dog will shake himself thoroughly and with enormous enthusiasm before completely stretching his whole body. All this movement ensures total contraction of the muscles; it gives them more elasticity, so that subsequently they relax more easily. Stretching actually elongates the muscles, which releases the blood and results in improved circulation. This is one of the basic principles of hatha yoga. The maximum contraction is obtained when breathing in and released when breathing out. Stretching not only unlocks the vertebrae but has a calming and tonic effect upon the nervous system. These muscular contractions, inhalations, temporary breath retentions, and exhalations restore normal breathing. This, in its turn, improves the circulation of the blood, which has a tendency to rush to the head during any intellectual activity. This point is more fully explained in the chapter on exercises.

2. Relaxation using the law of gravity

The muscles should be relaxed one after the other – the whole process being controlled by thought. This loosens up all the tense, contracted parts in one swoop. The first time round, confine exercise to observation of the muscles and their positions. Then, when the exercise is repeated, you must actually feel the muscles relaxing. The formula here is: *Look*, then *feel*.

3. Detached relaxation

This is particularly suitable for beginners, as it involves economy in the use only of the basic muscles.

While writing, use only the fingers, leaving both arm and hand quite limp. Open a door in the same way, hold a spoon, or shake hands – the principle is the same. An enormous amount of energy is saved.

4. Yoga relaxation explained

The key is breathing. Lie on the ground, in a state of detachment, then breathe in and breathe out as you 'leave' each part of the body. Make a systematic tour of the body, starting with the feet and working up to the head, including the skull and the brain inside it. Breath, muscles and brain all work in conjunction, and the reason is complementary. It might be supposed, that as this is common knowledge, they would not be allowed to go their own way, but unfrotunately, such is not the case in everyday life. The results are short, rapid breathing or breathlessness, and a mind wandering as aimlessly as though it had no connection with the body it is supposed to serve. This is anarchy. The body is a uniquely constructed mechanism which reacts to stimuli with either pain or pleasure. On the other hand, it is readily accepted that the brain, although uniquely individual, may be enslaved by friend or foe.

The intellect was created to serve a specific function, in direct proportion to that of the fingers or the legs. Just as a dog *possesses* a good nose, without actually *being* a good nose, man possesses a mind, but he is not the mind—which yogis compare to a mad monkey stung by a scorpion. The brain is capable of very grave errors, with disastrous results to the owner – at best, despair; at worst, suicide. But man can discover another dimension of himself outside his mind. It is one which will assist him in self-renewal, in the restoration of his sense of values, and in a general reconditioning and regeneration. The secret is relaxation. It effects a complete transformation, a positive orientation of life and events. Any change in a life-style automatically changes the reasons for any unfortunate consequences, and so eliminates them. Muscular and mental relaxation has brought responsibility and success to many, and yet it is available to all those who care to benefit from it.

This process or relaxing tensions, and unloading all extraneous mental activity, could be described as a kind of re-birth to, in a sense, the state of Adam as he was at the beginning, created by love. With the refreshment of the spirit, the presence of Jesus becomes a living reality, and the depths of one's being open up to receive God's word.

How does this control of the mind work? Indeed, directing the brain is no easy matter, but it is simplified when its closest collaborator – observation – is brought into action. A person who is always glancing nervously about is a familiar sight, and the conclusion is that he is probably worried. But he can help himself, if only he would realize it. First, he should keep still, and learn repose, then he could pause to admire a beautiful view, or any interesting aspect of his surroundings. In his own home he could provide himself with a sacred statue or image, such as Christ in all his glory. The presence of this would benefit him, and simply by gazing at it, he would be filled with joy. Then a smile of well-being would soon replace the worried frown!

The mind's other collaborator is breathing, a faithful servant, and although quite unobtrusive, at a word of command immediately capable of positive action. Breath is life. The preservation of life is considered to be of primary importance; breathing should be accorded similar care. Inhalation and exhalation play a most important part in relaxation for the purpose of prayer.

For a Christian, relaxation is the removal of a blindfold and the discovery of the light. It is a leave-taking, where all anxieties are rejected. It is a re-birth, where the new person has simply returned to his original state. Christ can now fill the being of this unfettered and unrestricted newborn child. For the baptized, relaxation means a joyous acceptance of death, transcendance, and resurrection in the divine presence. The pivot of all these relaxations is the unison of mind and breathing. With

13

each exhalation, the amalgamation of these two makes it just that much easier to relax the muscles, to unload all the garbage cluttering up the mind, and to wave anxieties good-bye. Breathing out is reununciation – unconditional surrender. This state creates a climate in which inspiration can flourish and renew the body, enabling the soul to reach out to God, and so receive strength.

An extraordinary number of tensions are nourished solely by greed. The practice of relaxation brings freedom from this vice. The body and soul are bared, and the heart is opened to God in a complete revelation of self in which there should be no shame, but rather joy: joy in being known, recognized, and illumined by the light of his countenance. His is the source of purification; he offers the promise of salvation from greed to those who do not shun him. To strip naked before God is to walk upon the path of purity and to approach perfect peace.

Each student should evolve his own personal method of relaxation, and discover its relation to prayer, based upon the stages described, which are the product of long personal experience.

(a) For me, the spiritual dimension of relaxation was first illustrated by the death and resurrection of Christ. Voluntary inactivity or immobility is a kind of temporary death, allowing Christ to accomplish his work, by increasing the awareness of his presence, and so bringing regeneration. Hence conscious immobility is a preparation for a true awareness of God.

(b) This stage leads to a wonderful experience – transparency. Just as a calm transparent lake will reflect the sky, so the practitioner of relaxation achieves a surface transparency which will reflect the image of God. Jesus's infinite pity does not hesitate; he is superimposed upon the poor human form with all his glory and strength. Although man is made in God's image, only surrender to Christ the Lord will remake man as the image of God.

(c) The third stage brings unity to mind and body by eliminating all internal duality. With a real sense of the collaboration between these two elements one's usual alienation may simply disappear. Human failure is all too often the result of the malfunction of the physical body. Only when the body performs correctly will the individual reach full potential.

(d) The last stage may cause some astonishment. There are those who will be startled, and even those who will be afraid. But revelation usually causes consternation. The divine regard has the power to pierce man through; disguise is useless, whether by dress or deception. The last stage, therefore, is nudity. Man must stand naked under the eyes of God, and be joyful in doing so, for he is presenting himself freely to love, and to inner purification. Now, the superficial transparency goes deeper, and permeates his being. He is inhabited by the light and the love of God; he has become more than just a mirror with a reflection. Just as the vine will bear delicious translucent grapes if it is planted where it can catch the sun, so is man renewed by the light of God's eyes. Each individual, according to the means at his disposal, is called to discover a tiny facet of the Father Creator. In so doing, he achieves a spiritual goal, and accepts responsibility before God. My nine-month period of relaxation gradually led to this illumination, to spiritual availability to God. Each one of us must find his own way of relaxation transcended by faith.

B. God does not like stiff-necked people

'I see that these are stiff-necked people. Now leave me, my anger is inflamed against them, and I shall destroy them' (Ex. 32.9)

Yahweh himself remarked upon the consequences of being stiff-necked. The stiff-necked are neither available nor adaptable, they are strangled by the contractions of the neck and the throat, by tension, and this prevents the heart from collaborating with the brain. The result is withdrawal – a crushed, cramped unreceptiveness. This shrivelled attitude is deaf to forgiveness, neither can it know surrender, nor true humility. It is quite immovable. How could it bend the head? Drop the chin upon the chest? Be submissive? When the neck area is completely free from all tension, then the face may be lifted up to the Father in love and gratitude.

A stiff neck is hardly conducive to prayer; the simple movement cannot be made. All energy is wasted by the nourishment of useless leeches on the shoulders. These take root easily on the throat, the neck, the face, the eys, and the jaws – they are contractions or tensions. A supple neck is of the utmost importance for yoga and prayer.

The chapter on exercises contains a very important series of simple movements. They set free all the necessary areas, and although the contractions will return during the course of everyday life, they will gradually be eliminated. Concentration, in conjunction with dissociated relaxation, will affect each movement of the necessary muscles during any activity.

The muscles of the face are often contracted because of nervousness. A few minutes of relaxation will correct this condition and in time, only a few seconds may be needed to remove facial tension before prayer.

An upright posture is very important in yoga and prayer. It has been aptly christened the 'resurrection' posture ("Yahweh lives, before whom I stand,' said Elijah, and it is impossible not to imagine the prophet accompanying these words with an appropriate suppliant attitude. To face God or one's neighbour in an upright position, is to be at his disposition, and to be available to execute his orders. Are not the angels always represented as upright, as about to set off upon some mission which he has commanded? Does not the word 'angel' mean 'envoy' or 'sent'? Ezekiel, having fallen face down upon the ground, was raised up to hear the voice and then to be sent to those who had rebelled against God (Ez. 2, I).

The upright posture takes advantage of the vertical structure of the body and allows the arms to be extended. One by one, the vertebrae fall into place, and the nerves behave appropriately. There must be an equilibrium between all parts of the body; only the right attitude can correct any imbalance in movement, or during any activity. A supple neck will give the correct position to the head, and walking will prove less tiring.

In traditional Hindu yoga, the upright posture is called 'Tadasana', which means 'a mountain'. Mountains are considered sacred, symbolizing as they do the reconciliation of earth and sky. In this posture, man identifies with a mountain, because of his solidity in relation to the ground. He must leap to answer the divine summons.

The Christian view of man is an upright one; it is the glory of the Father, it is Jesus appearing in the garden, it is Jesus saying again 'Leave me'. (Mark, 5,41; Luke, 7,4 and 8,54.) That is to say, 'Make yourselves upright, because I shall raise you up even as I do myself.'

II THE PILLAR OF FIRE AND THE HUMAN SPINAL COLUMN

'Yahweh led his people in the form of a column . . .' (Ex. 13, 21)

God, who has fashioned us in his image, manifests himself in the form of a column of cloud or fire, in order to guide his people through all their trials. The column represents life, progress and evolution. Sometimes it appears as a cloud, sometimes as fire, which is strangely similar to a force which the Hindus named Kundalini. This force is said to be able to mount the human vertebrae like a serpent of fire.

The spinal column has been called the tree of life, as it is a kind of trunk around which man is structured. The hollows of the vertebrae contain the 'fire of life', for this is where all human energy circulates, nourishing the muscles, nerves, plexus and so on. The two polarities, positive and negative, are represented by each side of the column, which in itself indicates the extreme importance of a correct posture. This should be supple, permitting these two forces to maintain a harmonious equilibrium. Any rigidity would make this impossible. The materiality and immateriality of the human being are extremely mysterious, a secret closely guarded by the vertebrae, with which it is inextricably linked. This merger of the physique and the psyche is the region where hatha yoga postures work progressively towards freedom.

God, manifested in the form of a column, said: 'I am the Living God', and similarly, man's spinal column is his life. Erected on the ground, it nevertheless reaches for the stars.

The spinal column is composed of five sacred vertebrae, which are joined together. There are five lumbar, twelve dorsal, and seven cervical vertebrae, and a fully comprehensive investigation into the human vertebrae would undoubtedly yield some interesting and illuminating information. The Great Mathematician creates nothing by chance, or by whim. However, the following are simply the results of basic practical investigations, but they are based upon experience.

The spinal cord is attached to the bulb of the coccyx, and it is protected by a flexible series of vertebrae. From between each vertebra springs a nerve fibre; these fibres nourish the ganglia of the nervous system. The organs, such as the heart, lungs, liver and stomach and so on, are protected by the plexus. Those who really wish to acquire a complete understanding of the infinite repercussions of the postures of hatha yoga should also study the mechanism of the human body. The modern sedentary life-style has an unpleasantly cramping effect, and because of this, the muscles of the back contract. The vertebrae, no longer supported, collapse one on top of the other, so that the nerve endings remain pinched just when they should be doing their job of providing regeneration and nourishment. Clearly, the vertebrae must be allowed their full potential, and the answer is stretching. This should be done very gently; absolutely no rough movement is required, just a routine of exercises which each individual should evolve for himself and his own needs. The back and the abdomen would also benefit from a 'remuscling' as they are intimately linked. Every hunched back has a corresponding corporation, and *vice versa!* This is a simple law of equilibrium. A round back contracts the shoulders, resulting in general 'sloth', so that the individual no longer benefits from the totality of his dynamism. This is partly because of the contractions of the shoulders, and partly because the diaphragm is blocked by the position of the body, so it loses its mobility. This 'come-and-go' facility of the diaphragm is supposed to relay and activate the internal organs. It affects the functioning of the lungs which take in oxygen and practical energy, and vitalizes the blood. The role of the blood is to clean, repair and regenerate all the living cells of the body. Here we have what amounts to a miniature interior workshop. This brief description should suffice to illustrate the lasting complementarity of the different elements of man.

Is there a really apt description for rounded shoulders and hunched backs? And what kind of instruction will correct the fault? Certainly not the old-fashioned command to 'keep yourself straight!' On the contrary, a child straightening up his back will almost immediately contract again, and the resulting collapse is a distressing sight. Some other, dependable solution, is required. A healthy back, without any deformity, will give the correct support, and this is where the lungs play their part, which is not just to force the wall of the thorax into a convenient position, but to open out the thoracic cage, which enables the lungs to settle themselves more comfortably so that they can carry out their work. It can be dangerous for those who are tense and contracted and have a tight chest to do breathing exercises. In order to give the body suppleness, mobility and muscular flexibility, follow the exercises in gymnastic yoga. Hatha yoga will restore suppleness and effect decontraction, but it is equally desirable that the muscles should be worked on, otherwise the ligaments will not function adequately. This is an important point. Perfect musculation gives access to many of the postures which are outside the scope of the average student, and Shri Mahesh, well-known for his work in the field, possesses a musculature which is a sheer marvel.

The hatha yoga postures used for prayer, and for the preparation for prayer, are precisely those which restore the suppleness of the back. This allows a proper articulation of the vertebrae, and facilitates the irrigation of the various organs of the body. Stretching has an excellent effect on the nervous system, as it fuses the physical, the mental, and the spiritual, at the exact point where they all meet. In view of this, be cautious; follow a carefully calculated method rather than any rough-and-ready approach. Work to a rhythm which reflects the laws of the universe – without any disorder. The body should be treated much as gardener tends his flowers, then the vertebral column will again be fully mobile. The key is gentleness.

During the first stage, it is advisable to begin by discovering all the articulations of the body, particularly those of the hips and the lumbar region. So many people waddle about like ducks! They simply have no idea how their parts articulate, and do not know how to find out. This is done quite simply by placing the hands on the hips and feeling the articulation roll under the fingers while rocking the body backwards and forwards. Feel something like a rocking motion in the region of the buttocks, while making sure that the lumbar region is supple and mobile. The lumbar region is the source of youth, and from it spring many dynamic qualities. Next, cross your arms, then, without sinking the chin on to the chest, bend down, feeling the articulation of the body at hip level, without hunching the back. This will relieve the pressure on the back. The following simple exercises are given in the appropriate chapter:

– stretching, in order to put the vertebrae back into place.
– massage, to activate the circulation.
– musculation, indispensible to the structure of the body.
– the harmonious development of the body, so that the lungs can settle down naturally into a desirable position. Harmonious movement is of the utmost importance, as this has profound repercussions upon the interior of the being. Avoid all jerky gestures.

III BREATHING AND LONGING FOR GOD

*'And the Lord God formed man of the dust of the ground,
and breathed into his nostrils the breath of life; and man
became a living soul' (Gen. 2, 7)*

Ever since God breathed the breath of life into the nostrils of man, life
has begun with an inhalation and ended on an exhalation. The breath of
God and the breath of life are intimately linked, and a number of biblical
texts testify to this:

'And all the while my breath is in me, and the Spirit of God is in my
nostrils' (Job 27, 3).

'The Spirit of God hath made me, and the breath of the Almighty hath
given me life' (Job 33, 4).

'If he set his heart upon man, if he gather unto himself his spirit and his
breath;
All flesh shall perish together, and man shall turn again unto dust' (Job
34, 14–15).

Man feels very profoundly that his breath comes from God; so much so,
that in all languages, breath and spirit are expressed by a single word.

Hindu yogis are all convinced that the Universal Spirit lives and
breathes in each thing and each being. With his last breath, a Westerner
'gives up the spirit' very much as an Oriental leaves his body after having
exhausted the number of respiratory cycles which had been accorded to
him at the moment of his birth. The life of a yogi is not measured in
days, but in a number of respiratory cycles. Yogis learn how to slow
down their breathing to a measured rhythm, which inevitably makes their
breathing better than that of the Occidental, who ignores the influence
of respiration upon each individual. There is no doubt that the quality of
breathing has a direct influence upon health, and in consequence upon
longevity.

Certain illnesses in which listlessness plays a large part have been the
subjects of many plays. Perhaps one of the most famous of the unhappy
heroines of these pieces was the Lady of the Camelias – but why did she
suffer as she did? It is now evident that the voluntary narrowing of the
thoracic cage, imposed by the fashion of the period, was responsible!

Short and rapid breathing indicates a nervous condition, whereas
measured breathing indicates a calm interior, and a better oxygenization
of the cells. Yogic respiration undoubtedly gives the best chance of
longevity. As respiration is life itself, it would be advisable for both
students and readers to take expert instruction before jumping in at the
deep end. Before practising certain breathing exercises, complete decontraction is absolutely essential. All the energy which is snuffed up and
expelled should circulate freely, and this process would be hampered by
tenseness. On a machine capable of reaching only a maximum of say 110,

the results of suddenly trying to rev it up to 220 would be disastrous! The real danger in yoga for Westerners is the spirit of competition. Civilization is geared to competition; it can do nothing without wanting to overdo it, an attitude which is totally incompatible with the relaxation and detachment of this discipline. Incidentally, a slight dizziness is not a particularly disturbing symptom to experience during breathing exercises, it is imply a sign that the blood is receiving some unaccustomed oxygenization.

The division of respiration into two parts creates a positive and a negative – inhalation is positive; toning the system, carrying oxygen to the lungs and providing the energy which the blood carries throughout the body. Exhalation is negative; purifying the body of carbon, which has a calming effect of great benefit during the posture exercises, as it allows the ligaments to relax and improves the suppleness of the body. Two aspects of yoga respiration require particular care and attention: every yoga exercise is composed of long spells of breath retention, and the ability of the lungs both to retain and expel breath is enormously increased. The lungs are encouraged to fill and empty more often and more thoroughly. Because of this, in the initial stages, a certain degree of discomfort in breathing could be experienced, and sometimes it takes about six months for the lungs to function normally and comfortably.

There are a number of obstacles to be overcome before good breathing can be acquired:

– the collapse of the back. This causes a slackening of the abdomen, so that the thoracic cage becomes so pinched that it is unable to budge.
– the reverse. When the shoulders and stomach are held like those of a soldier on parade, the work of the diaphragm is impeded.
– problems which affect the solar plexus in the pit of the stomach; fear, anguish, jealousy, and so on obstruct breathing.

The voice is improved by relaxation and breathing; the above-mentioned impediments are a direct hindrance to the good quality of the voice. The physical state may be assessed by the sound of the voice and the evolution of the whole personality depends upon good breathing. There is a bond between conscious respiration and responsibility. The centre of gravity (beneath the navel) is the source of happiness, putting man into contact with all the vital parts of his being and all the powerful forces which inhabit him, making him strong in the face of adversity, and giving him access to all the riches possessed by his inner self. And conscious respiration controls all this.

Even the very simple exercises which unclamp the diaphragm have brought serenity to a number of nervy students who have undertaken the course of exercises suggested in this work. They met life's difficulties of existence with much more equanimity and solved their problems more competently. They ceased to be upset by trivialities and became more lucid in their judgments.

The lung's collaborators

1. The arms

Hatha yoga exercises provide what is virtually a 'remission en route'. The prime mover here is complementarity; all the collabroators of the lungs are called upon for their participation, the first being the arms, which are a natural continuation of the lungs. The movement of the arms facilitates the functioning of the lungs, a point of which the beginner should be aware at all times. The Egyptians were certainly conscious of this when they practised the ancient art of twirling sticks, and it is for the same reason that 'lungs-arms' exercises are advised. Perhaps the best is that in which a heart is symbolically traced by the hands. As in most exercises, the movement ascends in the beginning on an inhalation of breath, while the descending movement is accompanied by an exhalation.

In order to clean out the lungs, it is very important to begin by exhaling rather than inhaling. It is unwise to top up the stale contents of a bottle with fresh liquid, and in the same way, inhaling before exhaling would merely be fouling the intake of fresh air. Of course, a little stale air is sure to remain in the lungs, but nevertheless, it is necessary to try to expel as much as possible in order to clean out the pulmonary cells.

However, do not inhale to the maximum, always leave a little space so that the exhalation may be controlled. Exhalation is slower, and twice as hard as inhalation. Certain exercises require that enough room for expansion be left in the lungs.

2. The diaphragm

The second collaborator of the lungs is the diaphragm, a powerful muscle which is found in the hollow of the stomach. It is of great importance to the functioning of the body in general, but particularly in view of its proximity to the digestive organs and the solar plexus, it is of immense value as far as the voice is concerned. Singers all know this, as it permits them to hold a note, and if it is blocked not only will the note waver and fall, but the voice will be flat. Vocal exercises aid remission in all respiration, and they provide a splendid form of relaxation. Onomatopoeia in the sung vowels on the scale (iii, aaa – etc.) will automatically activate the muscle. Great strides in this field have been made by Marie-Louise Aucher, the founder of psychophony in France. The way a singer's breathing projects the voice is different from the yoga method of respiration, which is more like the pschycophonic method. The singer uses the throat in a way that provokes a slight interior bruising, whereas the yoga respiration, like psychophony, concentrates on opening out the inner self. After all, whether the voice talks or sings, it is a means of communication – of opening out to others. The physical exercises suggested in this series are very simple, inoffensive, and within reach of all. Above all, the all, the diaphragm will not be able to resist them. They will not work miracles, but effort and perseverance will certainly be rewarded. In addition to the improvement of the respiratory functions, and all that they involve, the diaphragm uses a new and unaccustomed mobility to rally all the internal organs and improve the digestive system. In a later stage, a method of controlled respiration will be given. Indispensable to the fight against nerves, calm and regular breathing not only improves the health, but the psychic equilibrium. Of even greater significance is the creation of an inner calm which makes the whole being more receptive and flexible.

Activation of the diaphragm permits the completion of the whole process of exhalation and inhalation. As much breath as possible is expelled, and the intake is made absolutely naturally and spontaneously. Any blockage is gradually eliminated, and with this accomplished, the whole self may be brought into being. Little by little, the understanding develops that others may be liked without being possessed, and that any affection given should not depend upon the advantage or reward likely to be obtained in return. Finally, it is possible to approach the unconditional love of God; to discover the new covenant, which is directly derived from the surrender of Christ to the will of his Father. The profoundest feeling of all may now be experienced – the opening up and sharing of the heart with God.

The second part of this work includes some simple exercises which comprise a complete plan for yoga respiration.

Jean Déchanet gives a perfect explanation of the influences of respiration upon prayer: 'The benefits of rhythmical breathing are felt especially during prayer . . . because both body and soul are involved in a united effort. This phenomenon is really quite an ordinary and purely physical automatic law.'

Conscious respiration leads to meditation, which in its turn increases the desire for prayer and a longing for the divine presence of God.

IV THE POSTURES

A General features

A posture, or asana, is a position which the body is able to maintain effortlessly for some length of time. In India, a yogi does not claim mastery of an asana unless he is able to maintain it for three hours. Westerners are content to hold a posture for a few minutes! There are 8400 postures, but it is not necessary to know all of them. The basic postures suffice to avoid monotony; where some improvement seems desirable, variants may be substituted from time to time. Yogis have observed that in nature, particularly as far as animals are concerned, certain qualities are dominant in each species. Thus, most of the postures carry the name of an animal or a plant, as the divine plan is so perfect that each element has received a gift which is quite unique. The tortoise, for example, symbolizes the retreat of the senses, detachment, interiorization; whereas the tree, the posture of equilibrium, symbolizes stability. This work deals only with the fairly simple postures, and does not include acrobatic exploits. There is no doubt that the pose adopted by the body has profound interior repercussions, and by means of prayer, the body collaborates with the soul. The combination of the living prayer and the living body constitutes a total offering which makes it impossible for the mind to be alienated by parasitic thoughts and ideas. Prayer is an introduction to the symbolism of the body. This chapter deals with the fundamental objectives of the postures, which are valid for all hatha yoga postures. All may be practised from the point of view of prayer, or of simple physical health. The body is a marvellous instrument, but like any musical instrument, it responds well only to expert handling. The different elements of the body all have natural functions to perform, and natural *modus operandi*. Prayer does not preclude the use of skilled techniques in the attainment of the body's full potential. Experiments have shown that the postures are supported by prayer, while the same postures are much more difficult to manage when their purpose is simply to improve the health. For example, the theme of grace has a very beneficial effect upon the postures, but irreverent groups find some difficulty in achieving the greeting of the sun. But beginners who take their cue from this work on yoga and prayer will surely be guided towards the means of purification and a true awareness of God by learning natural respiration and so becoming part of the great universal harmony. Gradually, the intensity of the quality of prayer will be infinitely increased if the postures are carried out according to the instructions given. Many agile students tend to try to forge ahead too quickly, but they succeed in doing little more than reaching the level of a good gymnast. Gymnastics are a set of quick and repetitive movements which make great demands upon the visible muscles of the body. Hatha yoga is a complete discipline which concerns the totality of man – physical, mental and spiritual. The following important points should always be observed while carrying out any posture:

– although it is necessary to be conscious of the internal movements of the body, they should be allowed to glide into the position of the posture without any force. In fact, one does not carry out a posture at all; one carries oneself into a posture. Nor does one imitate a posture; one lives it internally.
– control all movement, but use as few muscles as possible. The others should be kept relaxed.
– be sure to keep the breathing smooth and controlled during the dynamic phase of the posture.
– allow the body to fall naturally into position. For example, in the plough posture, do not push the feet on to the ground; wait until they fall into place by means of their own weight. The same applies to the sitting postures (the lotus, or various simplifications); relax the knees and

wait until they descend of their own accord.

– do not be tense. If there is any difficulty in relaxing, think beautiful thoughts. No force should be used; relax, loosen thoroughly, and exhale.

– learn how to extend the length of time a posture may be held. For example, the twist on exhalation, which relaxes the ligaments. Always remain still during inhalation.

– to maintain an acquired posture, relax the body again, and breathe in and out regularly and evenly. Any blockage of the breath is not advised. Allow the muscles to stretch out and work without blood; these first moments can often be most arduous, but the reflexes soon become calmer, and absolute relaxation is possible. All concentration should be centred upon the breathing, as the posture is determined by the ventilating action of the lungs which is giving harmony to the body. Some schools will stress the importance of concentrating upon the particular organ concerned in the posture – kidnyes or glands, and so on. It is during this period that internal physiological reactions are produced which have no relation to gymnastics; it is the period when prayer, its theme oriented by the position of the body, is born and begins to blossom.

– to leave the posture, maintain perfect control. Do not make any jerky movements, as the body is still working to find and keep the universal harmonious rhythm which helps you return to the same posture. On descending from the plough, it should be possible to feel all the vertebrae place themselves one by one on the ground, and it is essential that the body should be spread out entirely on the ground, relaxed by its own weight. These few seconds are complementary to the posture as they allow it to take effect. The muscles are brought back to normal by the flow of blood which has been oxygenated by the slow and regular breathing during the posture. Not only are the muscles invigorated, but there is an improvement in energy, as when the body has been permeated by a posture, the meridians are activated. All that remains is for all this process to effect the transformation – calm and relaxation will reign, and with this return to the natural order of things, nature herself is able to restore the equilibrium. The greatest beneficiaries of the postures are perhaps the endocrine glands. Their position in the body rather resembles that of a group of planets, and their work is of tremendous importance. The pituitary gland, which is the 'leader' of the group, is oxygenated and kept in trim by slow deep breathing. The other glands are either stretched out or contracted during the postures, constituting something like a series of internal 'massages', after which they should be allowed to rest.

The intervals between the postures may be spent very profitably forming the appropriate prayers. During this time it is likely that certain verses from the Psalms will spring to the minds of some students. Psalm 23 contains the verse which probably comes to mind first – 'He maketh me to lie down in green pastures . . .' This quotation perfectly describes the sense of release felt after a posture.

Before undertaking the following postures, deep breathing and stretching are advised. Also, it is preferable that the order of the postures should be carefully selected, so that the movement and gestures of one lead naturally into the movement and gestures of the next. Thus, all useless activity is eliminated, and an even flow maintained.

The following categories of postures are illustrated in a later section.

– The postures of the back:

These make the spinal column supple, so that from the nape of the neck to the coccyx it becomes more and more mobile as the work progresses, and the soothing effect takes place. The polarity is negative. (closed postures: E 11, 13, 14 – G26, 27, 28, 29, 30: J39)

– The postures of the stomach:

The abdominal region is supported by inhalation, which has a toning effect. The polarity is positive (open postures, not to be done before sleeping: F 16–25).

– The postures of the torso:

There are numerous postures of the torso, a soothing effect being achieved by a supine posture (h32), and a toning effect by a sitting or upright posture (H31). Both supine and upright postures are of great physiological benefit because they preserve the flexibility of the lumbar region, which is the source of youth. Equally, they facilitate the work of the meridian circling the waist, and as this is instrumental in changing polarities, body energy is affected. Abstention from sex is recommended after these postures.

– The upright postures:

These involve the articulation of the hips, the knees, and the muscles of the thighs; they also produce maximum aeration of the lungs (e.g., the triangle: B38).

– The reversed postures:

These are either positive and soothing (the candle, E12) or negative and bracing (the pear tree). Here the polarities are reversed, the body recharging itself positively through the soles of the feet, instead of the negative attraction of the feet to the earth. There is also an effect upon the circulation of the blood and the lymphatic system. In contrast to some methods, hatha yoga does not advise the lengthy maintenance of these postures.

– The postures of equilibrium:

These are numerous (I 33–37), the tree, the frog and the eagle being the simplest and most adaptable for the purpose of prayer. They demand stability while simultaneously all the parts of the body are relaxed; they promote concentration, facilitating co-ordination and interiorization; physiologically they correct any faults in the spinal column; they have a beneficial effect upon the pituitary gland, co-ordination, and the cerebellum; they provide mental equilibrium, which is necessary for the integration of the personality and the establishment of an ordered mind. In restoring the equilibrium of the container, the contents are also restored!

Except for the posture of the head, which is bracing, all these postures are soothing, and considered suitable for everyone, including children and the aged. At first, it is permissible to cheat a little and occasionally use the wall as a prop while practising the sequence!
– The sitting postures:
These really come under the heading of postures of balance (J41–45).

B. A complete Hatha Yoga programme

This programme is composed of a number of stages; they include the following exercises:

1. Preparation: purifying exhalations while the body is kept quite still and completely relaxed 'See Series A).
2. Stretching and warming up (See Series B).
3. A closed posture – on the knees, or sitting (See Series C).
4. The work of the abdominals – on the back (See series D).
5. A reversed posture – the candle or the chariot (See series E).
6. An open posture – on the back, like a fish; on the stomach, like a cobra, grasshopper, or bow (See series F).
7. A closed posture – like a pair of pliers, or a bent leaf (See series G).
8. The torso (See series H).
9. Breathing, followed by resting on the ground.
10. The postures of balance. (See series I).
11. Relaxation (Fig. 1, 2, 3).

Between numbers 9 and 10, some upright postures may be carried out, but never interpose the reverse postures, as they should be done only in the middle of the sequence, or as a conclusion. Between each posture some time should be allowed for relaxation.

Before starting the chariot type postures, the spinal column should be made more supple and flexible, but it should be borne in mind that no forcing is necessary. The back, and indeed, the whole body, should be prepared gradually, so that little by little all the elements co-ordinate and fall naturally into the posture. For example, before beginning the 'pliers', some work on the articulation of the hips is usually necessary.

Stretch, elongating the body as much as possible. Raise the chest higher than usual, then place the hands on either side of the body, lowering the chest, while articulating at hip level. Now raise the body, not by the heels and hands, but on an inhalation. Return to the sitting position, then lengthen out on an exhalation. Make a V-shape with the legs, and place one foot against the opposite thigh, then lower the body, so that the chin touches the knee. With the legs placed tailor-fashion, do the same movements. In these positions, or in the half-lotus, articulate the hips, trying to touch the ground with the chin. Change the position of the arms, crossing them behind the back, on each side of the body.

Before undertaking the chariot: raise the legs, one after the other, bend, then straighten out. The abdominal region should always be exercised thoroughly before this posture. Sit up, so that the lumbar region is resting completely flat on the ground.

For the open postures of the cobra type: gradually straighten up the spinal column by modifying the position of the arms: in front; at the sides; bent; straight; crossed behind the back, and so on. After a closed posture of the folded leaf type, this will replace the vertebrae and relax the back.

As far as the torso is concerned, it is advisable to stretch out on the ground before taking the sitting position, as this will have a soothing effect.

Open postures increase energy, while closed postures (such as the pliers) produce calm. Most of the 84,000 postures may be modified or replaced where it seems necessary or desirable to the individual, but an open posture is interchangeable only with another open posture, and so on: e.g., the fish replaced by the diamond or the hero, the pliers replaced by the tortoise.

The hatha yoga postures should never be confused with gymnastic exercises; they have totally different goals. The object of an asana is clear-cut and single-minded, and may best be summed up as follows:

(a) to condition the physical body so that it may easily absorb the flow of spiritual energy, which will increase awareness. The mind is controlled through the will and, after the period of preparation, the mind is no longer adversely affected by a malfunctioning body.

(b) to find stability and immobility; all movement ceases, but there is no rigidity.

(c) Initially, it may be found that a great deal of effort is required in order to keep a position for any length of time. Mental consciousness is mobilized by stillness of the body, so subsequently, the posture is held correctly by the body by means of the unconscious mind. It is the 'release of effort', to quote the Sutras of Patanjali, II, 47. Practice of the asanas must always precede that of the pranayamas. The postures develop and strengthen the will-power, as well as spiritual energy.

A number of the postures listed are described as 'praying' postures, and many types of postures have the theme of grace. The immobility and surrender of the body into one attitude or another makes the body receptive to the state of prayer, both encouraging and nourishing it.

Essentially, the whole point of this work is to illustrate physical participation in preparation for prayer.

Sessions should be organized in a style which is harmonious with the cycles of the seasons. For example, Advent would lend itself very aptly to a stripping of the interior during all meditation, relaxations, and postures. This would be in imitation of the vegetation at this period, which strips itself of all ornament, and stands revealed in total nudity. Similarly, every inner burden which does not conform to the image of

Christ should be rejected. This is also a period of waiting: waiting for the Saviour – for nature – for renewal. Equally, it is a period of hope – hope that the grain will germinate in the earth – that the dead leaves will form a humus to nourish the sap of the future tree. For the process or renewal is inextricably linked to the laying bare of renunciation. Yoga and prayer are a preparation for a new life.

C. THE SITTING POSTURE

'I will sit in the shadow of the Beloved'

There is an ever-increasing need in Man for divine love, a love which can be fulfilled by literally sitting in the shadow of the Beloved, and so becoming reunited with God through prayer. A sitting posture is ideally suited to this purpose as the body is, in effect, stablized by the ground and nourished by its contact with the earth. This helps to liberate the soul, which, although it has noble aspirations, must be free before it can soar to higher levels. Jean Déchanet, during sessions at Valjouffrey, practised a number of symbolic postures sitting on the ground, and this has since proved to be an adaptation most conducive to prayer.

To be seated on the ground is to be at the feet of Jesus; to abolish all material barriers between man and the Lord; to become a supplicant for his love. When a group offers up prayers together, each individual experiences the feeling of being a child again – a child in the company of other children of the same Father. The sitting posture is a posture of humility; there is a voluntary renunciation of mobility. Jesus made the crowd sit, not simply out of courtesy, but so that they would be able to concentrate fully upon his teaching and his miracles. An example of this is surely the feeding of the five thousand. The yogis of India are trained with particular care in this position, because the advantages are numerous. Those which seem most appropriate in relation to prayer have been selected for inclusion in this work.

1. Good control of the spinal column is obtained by sitting on the ground cross-legged. The weight of the body being on the buttocks, the column is free and flexible, which liberates the abdomen and the diaphragm.

2. The diaphragm is now able to operate in the right way, and this facilitates respiration.

3. Respiration increases oxygenization of the lungs, and thus there is an improvement in the performance of the brain. While the legs are crossed, the circuit is closed and there can be no dissipation of energy. With the circulation temporarily closed down no unnecessary demands are made upon the blood supply.

4. In this position it is much easier to control the abdominal muscles. Respiration may now be practised according to the most advanced principles of yoga and zen techniques, and meditation is facilitated. In the

stretched out position there is always the risk of falling asleep, whereas from the sitting position all the attention may be devoted to tapping the sources which life offers. As the body has been rearranged in the minimum space, the centre of gravity is more easily accessible, transforming the sitting posture to a posture of equilibrium, which carries many attendant advantages.

5. From an immediate and practical point of view, this posture permits the conservation or recuperation of the knees, hips and so on, because there is an immense improvement in articulation. In consequence, suppleness is restored, and after all, suppleness is the surest possible guarantee of a youthful physique and mentality! It is to be expected that the first steps will prove to be the most difficult, as articulation (particularly of the thigh muscles) has probably atrophied. But this should not daunt anyone, as it is quite simply the result of sitting in chairs. So let the children sit on the floor. Of course, eventually even adults find that they are able to sit on the floor quite comfortably and naturally – but patience and a certain amount of caution are required. On no account should any force be used; gravity will do all the work. Relax and slacken the muscles whenever settline down on thick cushions, reclining in deep seats, or even pushing drawers back in with the rear end! In the chapter on exercises there is a simple design for a small seat which could be made by any carpenter, and which would certainly help articulation if it were to be used regularly.

Sitting on the ground has many variations, the main ones being the lotus and the half-lotus, for which some expertise is required. The Carmelite posture is a sitting posture, but on the heels. The preparatory techniques for these postures are in series J.

II PREPARATORY EXERCISES

INTRODUCTION

The discipline of yoga requires a strict adherence to a programme of precise preparatory exercises. Those who are anxious to try the postures should never allow their impatience to cause any neglect of these exercises. Impatience is contrary to the discipline itself, which demands complete detachment from any idea of attainment, achievement, or result. One does not do yoga, one enters into it. Some see yoga as a series of set contortions performed on a mat for a certain length of time, which would invariably prove to be strenuous. Yoga is intended as an alternative way of life – a more authentic and profound way of life. The postures provide the verification of an interior state, neither their number nor their complexity constituting much importance. The essential aspect is the fashion in which the postures are lived; a visible application of the control and surrender of the postures permanently made manifest in the complete life-style.

Traditional yoga is composed of eight stages which lead the expert into the discipline. The first two (yama and niyama) precede the asanas, which are third. Yama and niyama are the stages of purification.

Yama means non-violence, truth, honesty, continence, and non-covetousness.

Niyama concerns personal habits, such as the purity of the body, nutrition, contentment, and austerity – all of which, through a knowledge of self, lead to the discovery and knowledge of God, and to his Scriptures, so leading also to a greater devotion to him.

The asanas concern breath control, which prepares the body for all the following stages, which are meditative, and represent union with God.

Most Westerners jump in at the deep end when they begin to study yoga. Bravely, they almost hurl themselves at the postures, without any previous preparation, and with absolutely no intention of changing their mode of existence or current life-style. This is more serious than it might at first appear, because modern life provokes and creates aggressions in man.

A certain physical preparation therefore is indispensable, and this section is devoted to exercises in preparation for yoga. They are planned to facilitate the entry into yoga, and will do so, providing that they are carried out without any spirit of competition. The postures themselves should not be attempted until the following objectives have been achieved:

1. Reconstruction of the back by balancing the spinal column (B 6 and 7).

2. Stretching, and feeling the movement and co-ordination of the muscles.

3. Relaxing the body: on the back; at the sides; on the stomach (A 1, 2 and 3).

Using breathing to relax the body, and making it supple, not by repeated assaults, but by the surrender of the whole being. Physically, the muscles and nerves relax, the mind is at peace, and the whole being is available to God.

4. Preparing for meditation by stretching the face and the nape of the neck. Decontracting the eyes; pausing for the purpose of observing; listening to the 'humming' in the throat; restoring the equilibrium of the body, and rediscovering the centre of gravity.

5. Noticing and controlling respiration, and unblocking the diaphragm, so that it recovers mobility. Adopting rhythmic yoga respiration.

6. Freeing and setting in motion the vital energies of the body, by making the articulation more supple.

7. Making the legs more supple, in preparation for the sitting-on-the-ground postures.

8. Taking care of the body when it is mobile, and preparing it for immobility during the postures.

A. Rebuilding the back

1. The first step is relaxation. Let the shoulders fall, breathe out gently, with complete surrender, then raise the arms on an inhalation. Arms in the air, stretch to the maximum, and hook the thumbs together, in order to affect both sides of the spinal column. Then, very gently, lower the head, the arms, the shoulders, the torso – all on a slow exhalation. Allow everything to fall relaxed, as though stretching then releasing a rag doll. Lift the head back, swing the arms. Feel the vertebrae falling naturally back into place; be conscious of the reconstruction of the back. Replace the head, and repeat three times. This exercise will assist in a preliminary conditioning of the body, almost like the greetings exchanged at a first

introduction. Each inhalation becomes a gesture of praise, while each exhalation expresses thankfulness and humility. The head is held back in total surrender. The benefits are both mental and physical – the back is gently massaged and able to put energies into motion, and the contractions of the shoulders and nape of the neck enjoy their first experience of liberation. There is a sensation of warmth in the back, and a general sensation of well-being (B 6 and 7).

2. Lie stretched out lengthwise on a hard surface. Bend the legs and move the head a little so that the knees and the chin touch. If possible, maintain the position for a few minutes, feeling how the back is completely laid down on the ground. Breathe calmly and naturally. This attitude is helpful in cases of back problems, as it restores the nerve endings.

3. Easily and quickly, learn how to reconstruct the back in a sitting position, preferably on the heels, but a small bench or chair would serve the purpose equally well. At the level of the hips, rock the body so that it is lowered on an exhalation and raised on an inhalation. Be aware of the articulation on the ascent and descent, and also be conscious of the reconstruction of the back.

This exercise is finally completed by prayer, for the purification of the descent and the general toning and conditioning effects of the conscious rhythmic respiration lead naturally and directly to a state of mind and body which is conducive to prayer. The breath of God, given by him to man, if used in the right way, will surely lead man back to him. It is, after all, breath which keeps man upright and gives him life.

B. Stretching, toning and conditioning the muscles

1. Sit on the heels, and with fists thrust into the armpits, on an inhalation, describe circles with the elbows. The exhalation will bring freedom from tension in the areas affected by the movement. It is most important that the breathing should be regular and controlled.

2. Stand upright on one leg, then on the other, gradually learning how to use the position for decontraction. Then, balanced on both legs, raise the arms on an inhalation. On an exhalation, stretch to the maximum, then with both hands, hold up imaginary walls to right and left. This exercise develops the thoracic cage and conditions the pulmonary system, transforming a skimpy F2 into a comfortable F5, and toning the back muscles, which are then able to do their job of holding up the vertebrae. It is quite clear that all the elements of the body are immutably linked, one to the other, and this produces a chain reaction, so of course, one deficiency causes another. Obviously, a back with well toned muscles is responsible for the good position of the body, which is an absolute

necessity for the supremely important respiratory system, as otherwise it cannot function adequately. Continue the exercise, remembering to exhale thoroughly, so that the back is fully stretched.

3. (a) The following exercise tones up the chest muscles. Lie on the back, legs apart, forming a St Andrew's cross. Raise the arms and legs alternately on an inhalation, then lower them slowly on an exhalation. Raise the limbs to a count of three; lower them to a count of six.

(b) Bend the legs, first right, then left, touching the forehead first with one knee then the other, then with both knees together.

(c) Sit cross-legged, first right, then left, touching the forehead first with one knee then the other, then with both knees together.

(c) Sit cross-legged, hugging the knees with the arms, then imitate a rocking-horse, co-ordinating the rhythm of the movements with the breathing. Rock forward – exhale; rock backward – inhale; controlling the whole depth of the middle of the back. Then, supported alternately first by one hand, then the other, similarly control each side of the back. Bend the legs, feet flat on the ground. Rest.

(d) Arms hugging the knees, roll on to each side to control and assemble all parts of the back. Bend the legs again, then turn on to the stomach.

4. The following exercise will tone up the back muscles. At first, work diagonally.

(a) Spread out to form a St Andrew's cross, inhale, raising a leg and an arm, then on an exhalation, lower them slowly. Raise to a count of three, lower to a count of six.

(b) Catch the left leg with the right hand, and *vice versa*.

(c) Raise the arms only, then the legs, then all four limbs simultaneously. This is a balancing movement. Touch the ground with the hands while the legs are raised, and *vice versa*.

(d) It is equally important to practise the classic exercise 'pumps', using the yoga respiratory method. Synchronize breathing and movement, rising on an inhalation to a count of three, and lowering on an exhalation to a count of six.

C. Relaxing the body

Whatever position the body takes, it must be relaxed. This applies at all times. To clarify:

On the back, on the sides, on the stomach: so that the really knotted areas may be unravelled. An unquiet mind is a source of tension, but a relaxed mind produces quite different reactions. At first, it is better to treat contractions as purely physical mechanisms, in order to prepare the way for a thorough spring-clean.

1. Muscular and mechanical relaxation

Lie on the back.

(*a*) On an inhalation, contract the entire body to the maximum, slowly raising the head and the limbs. Exhale, completely relaxing on to the ground. Repeat several times.

(*b*) Turn over on to the stomach.

Similarly, breathe in, contract to the maximum, and with fists clenched, first raise the limbs, then lower them. Stretch. Hook the thumbs together, control the balance, then release.

Do not attempt to undertake the following exercises during the initial stages; work up to them gradually.

The contractions and relaxations activate a healthy circulation, conditioning the lymphatic system and producing energy. They may be used in everyday life, during all occupations and activities.

The following exercise has acquired the nickname of 'puff pastry', as the body becomes a rolling pin! The solar plexus, centre of the emotions, is completely controlled.

(*c*) Lie on the stomach, arms lengthwise, head set evenly on the shoulders. The feet are apart, at about the width of the shoulders, hooked to the ground by the big toes, which are bent. Hands are flat, one on top of the other. Roll to left and right, the breathing being synchronised with each movement. Do not hurry; the pace should be measured. Keep both feet and hands fixed.

2. Relaxation on an immobile back (A1)

Lie on the back.

Be aware of the body; it should be completely relaxed. Settle the body, then restore the balance of the body, around an axis from the bridge of the nose to the navel. Surrender to the law of gravity; let the body go, it should not be held in any way. A raised limb should fall back on to the ground inert, without resistance. Allow the muscles to succumb to the magnetic pull of the earth, for she is the mother of nourishment. The earth affects all tensions and irritations, absorbing them into her bosom – but she can do this only if she is allowed to do so. This surrender of the body is a preliminary to a sweeping out of the mind.

(*a*) First, the face should be lit up by a smile, the lips relaxed, and the jaws loosened as much as possible. A Christian will recollect the radiance of the face on any statue of the Virgin Mary, with the arms gently held out in a gesture of welcome. Even the palms are opened out towards the sky – nothing is closed; nothing is closed out.

The feet are apart, pointed outwards, and quite unencumbered by the weight of the body. Legs, calves, knees, backs of knees, thighs, buttocks, pelvis, the whole of the back, shoulders, and the nape of the neck – all are eventually quite flat on the ground. Be conscious of the decontraction, the freedom, the untrammelled quality of each part of the body.

(*b*) During this second unloading of thought, observe the position and condition of the body.

(*c*) During the third stage, be aware of the volume of the body, dividing it up, from the feet to the head, including the contents of the cranium.

(*d*) Make a tour of the body, be aware of the body. Beginning with the heels, be conscious of each segment of the body and its contact with the earth.

At first, be content with stages (*a*) and (*b*), then experiment with (*c*) and (*d*) after a period of training. After exercising, manipulate the fingers and feet very slowly, stretch, yawn, roll from side to side, making the transition from immobility to activity very gently. For a short spell, avoid conversation.

3. Relaxation on the sides (A2)

Relaxation may be effected equally well while lying on the side, as in the position of a sleeping child. The head rests on the arms, or on one arm, with the other flung back. One leg is slightly bent. It is essential that the nape of the neck and the small of the back are loose. With arms bent, palm to palm under the head, use the breathing to relax the sides by exhaling while moving an arm to the hip. Move it back on an inhalation, then change sides. Be aware of the movement at the sides.

4. Relaxation flat on the stomach (A3)

The arms are bent as much as possible in front of the head, the hands one on top of the other, the forehead supported by the wrist, the chin poised on the ground. Thoroughly relax the nape of the neck. The feet may be pointed either inwards or outwards. Relax the back completely, thoroughly sweeping out the mind. Start at the coccyx and progress to the nape of the neck. Be aware of the vertebrae, and of the life which they protect; life which was freely given by God. The spinal column is a supple and precious part of that life, so it should be groomed meticulously. All the vital energies are kept by the spinal column, and they condition all aspects of life, including prayer.

In yoga and prayer it will be found that a certain position of the body is used as a position of humility and total surrender to the divine will. The back first being relaxed, the arms are placed in a cross, an attitude which has profound interior repercussions, and which, for good reason, has been selected as being ideally suited to ordinations.

5. Yoga relaxation, using the breath

True yoga relaxation uses the breath so that exhalation will relax the body and help muscular and mental surrender.

Lie stretched out on the ground, perfectly relaxed, completely surrendered to the pull of gravity, and with reference to all the principles of the first immobile relaxation. On each exhalation, move and thoroughly loosen each part of the body, right down to the feet. Then progress back towards the head. Do not forget to relax the arms, and each palm and every finger. This will produce a sensation of drowsiness, as the body will be first decontracted, then liberated. It is possible that the feeling of lightness and absolute availability will prove an excellent permanent beginning to a programme.

The St Andrew's cross has played a fairly prominent part thus far, and will further augment the opening exercises by completely loosening the solar plexus, which recharges itself with divine energy. Complete concentration upon this attitude will promote complete surrender, bringing an intensity of awareness to the state of prayer, the body having been purged of all desire for movement. In all relaxation, even that unrelated to prayer, be vigilant rather than somnolent, for fundamentally, the body should not be at all exhausted.

For a Christian, relaxation represents the death and resurrection of Christ. The exhalation phase corresponds to death voluntarily accepted as a purification and laying bare. Inhalation is a promise and an offer of rebirth after each surrender, during which the life of Christ is affirmed and strengthened. This total communion with the Lord can only come to those who are in a state of availability, and if the state of relaxation has been fully understood, and a sense of the parallel dimension experienced. Those who are religiously active, but too physically exhausted to be able to pray usually find a solution to the problem in this method of relaxation. It allows them to devote their lives entirely to God and to be motivated by the divine force, so that their evangelical duties may be undertaken in a spirit of joy. The prayers included in this work were all created during the course of relaxation. It will soon become apparent that all students may similarly learn to live their lives in the services of others by realising the bond between the position of the body and the deepest aspirations of the soul.

D. Preparing for meditation

Muscular relaxation is closely linked to mental relaxation and regular breathing. Mental relaxation is directly associated with observation, and all mental incapacity caused by agitation may be calmed by the posture of observation. This is one of the reasons why the postures of equilibrium are so strongly recommended for such cases. It is impossible to maintain the postures unless the observation is calmly concentrated upon a certain object. It is easy to relax the limbs as they are composed of a relatively small number of large muscles, but such is not the case with the face, where the eyes use a number of small muscles, and all agressions gather and establish themselves. In view of this, the relaxation of the face requires particular attention, and the following exercises were designed for this purpose.

1. Relaxation of the face

The lips must be relaxed and apart, the tongue should be limp and loose, the chin slack, the jaws unclenched, the forehead smooth, the eyelids fall naturally on the eyes, and the nostrils are relaxed.

2. Liberation of the neck, and the nape of the neck

The decontraction of the neck is no less essential. Sit down comfortably on the ground, taking a nun's position, with the hands resting on the knees. If sitting on the ground should present any difficulties, sit on a chair, or stand upright. Breathe out, and turn the head as far as possible over the shoulder, then gently bring the head back while breathing in. Turn the head to the other side, and breathe out, etc. This is one of the first yoga exercises, and it is unfortunate that modern life makes it impossible to use the exercise constantly. Believers, remember – God does not love a stiff neck! So making the neck supple is a first priority, and in the following simple exercise there should be a complete awareness of all movement, and the infinite repercussions should be experienced at the deepest level. The result will be a state which is receptive both to the word of God, and to all communication with the brotherhood of man.

If an occasional creak should be audible during the course of the exercise, breathe out, as this will bring a greater degree of relaxation. Always be gentle, never use force. After describing circles with the head, keep the mouth open and turn slowly on an inhalation, then when the chin touches the chest, turn on an exhalation. Should the nape of the neck prove to be very fragile, support it with the hands. Above all, make no attempt to rush things, prolong the periods gradually at a very controlled pace. Small doses are preferable to an excess! The contractions will become more and more superficial, until finally they will disappear altogether.

3. Decontracting the eyes

The eys are literally martyrs to everyday active life because they are absolutely forced to hold a fixed position for reading and writing at a short distance. This diminution of the field of vision not only weakens the vision, but also creates tensions. It has been established that outstanding improvements in vision can result from the following exercises, where the body in general, and the face in particular are relaxed. Before beginning the exercise, remember to remove your spectacles.

1. Look up to the left, then down; look up to the right, then down (repeat several times).
2. Turn the eyes up to the left, then down to the right, and *vice versa*.
3. Rotate the eyes in a circular motion.
4. Fix the eyes on the end of the nose, then turn them to peer as far away into the distance as possible (preferably at a beautiful view).
5. Enlarge the field of vision as much as possible, trying to notice everything of which the surroundings are composed. Tired eyes may be pleasantly soothed by resting them in the warm palms of the hands, the gesture itself having restful connotations.

4. The position of observation

The ground having been well-prepared, the position of observation should present no problems. The Christian particularly will find that the way to prayer has been opened up, and that he can make his way smoothly and with renewed strength.

Take up a comfortable sitting position, making sure that the face is perfectly relaxed. The beauties of the countryside provide excellent subjects for any outdoor observation, while such objects as statues of saints are suitable for indoor contemplative observation. At home, the statue should be placed a short distance away, within easy view. Complete relaxation and surrender should accompany the calm observation, when the meditative orientation will almost literally become a prayer. Observations of a similar nature were frequently made by Jesus himself:
Jesus beholding him, loved him . . . (Mark 10, 21).
Jesus looked round about . . .
But when he saw the multitudes, he was filled with compassion . . . (Mat 9.36).
Jesus lifted up his eyes and saw a great company . . . (John 6, 5).
And when Jesus beheld him, he said 'You are Simon' . . . (John 1, 42).
And the Lord turned, and looked upon Peter . . . (Luke 22, 61).

It is impossible not to feel the intensity of the way in which the Lord looked at Peter after his denial. Such a look takes in the whole being, and a Christian will have experienced the effects of all the looks of divine love which have been cast in his direction at different times, just as the resurrection of Jesus was experienced by Mary Magdalen in the garden, and by the gathering at Emmaus. The profound experience of feeling the divine glance must be created anew, so that may himself may regard his brother with the same compassion. The tenderness of Jesus and intensity of his love are perceptible in the calm of his regard, which gradually permeates man, and again fills him with love and tenderness for the whole of mankind.

Opening out and surrendering will transport the believer into prayer; prayer will virtually offer iteself up of its own accord! These spontaneous prayers are undoubtedly the most precious, and will surely lead to a greater awareness of the divine presence.

5. Listening to glottal humming

Glottal humming is produced by the friction caused when air passes deep down at the back of the throat. To listen to this humming aids meditation.

The chin points towards the sternum, the nape of the neck is perfectly relaxed. 'Interiorize' through the nostrils (this will involve slight sniffing), then close the eys and allow all thoughts to follow the path of the air through the throat. A slight humming, outwardly inaudible will then be heard internally. Now thread the mind into the noise, much as cotton is threaded into the eye of a needle. Allow the breathing to modify itself, but on each inhalation and exhalation, remain aware and fully conscious of being – of existing at the present moment.

6. The equilibrium of the body

The balance of the body is controlled by an invisible line which runs from the bridge of the nose to the navel. Observe the equality of both sides of the body. The sitting on the ground posture is a posture of balance, and all the postures of equilibrium facilitate the rallying and gathering together of all the energies of the body.

7. Hara, centre of gravity

When a state of stability and being present has been established, maintain it, allowing all thoughts to descend to a point under the navel. Feel the resistance of the descent of the diaphragm during the respiratory movements, then allow the breath to remount spontaneously, making the whole being blossom gloriously and pulsate with new life. In order to launch the total self towards divinity, that self must descend to the furthest depths of inner being.

The entrails of man correspond to the source of life, which in its turn is synonymous with the concept of 'mother', and the accompanying qualities of tenderness and compassion. At the emotional level, compassion inhabits the entrails – St Paul referred to 'compassionate entrails', and the Old Testament constantly represents Yahweh as a God with entrails, which may be interpreted as a God of love. For a Christian, love is the greatest force in the world, the Creator of all things created Man with love, and God never ceases to follow man with his love. He chose the entrails of a young girl as a means of giving his Son to the world, and in doing so, he made little Mary the mother of all men. For Christians, a conscious concentration on hara will produce transcendence. This miraculous passage of self through the entrails – through the cells of God – of Mary – and of the earth – is a resurrection of self. The centrifugal force of hara restores man to the centre of gravity, and the rebirth of the Christian brings a trenscendence which fully experiences the inexhaustible tenderness of God.

8. The body-mind tandem

The duality of body and mind is a constant source of suffering; an imbalance which leads to obsessions of all kinds. Any meditation or prayer will prove more fruitful when the mind is not at odds with the body. Absolute concentration upon any work or activity will automatically bring about a good balance between mind and body. Bad health and exhaustion are the results of mental anguish and a wandering mind, whereas the communion of mind and body will bring true peace, bringing man nearer to a real union with God.

When Adam saw Eve he cried: 'This is now bone of my bones, and flesh of my flesh! (Gen. 2, 23). He recognized the unity, the making of one flesh, which was a rejection of all covetousness. And covetousness is tension.

The offering of the self to God entails the reassembly of all available elements. Nothing should be neglected – there are no exceptions, because there must be no imbalance. The availability and transparency of God are hardly likely to be found where there is disharmony or friction. Body and mind must meet and unite – not only with each other, but with the self. This collaboration must be so complete that it resembles the consummation of love between husband and wife; different parts of the same whole are individually identifiable, yet linked. Only then can the mind and the body, like husband and wife, be fruitful according to the Will of the Father. This mind-body partnership must learn to relax together, have confidence in each other, and surrender themselves to each other in an intimate relationship where one literally becomes the other. All tension must be eliminated, so must all unhealthy complicity. This is a valuable universal law of love between spouses, and so it is with the mind-body relationship. Only this unity can bestow the power to rejoin the infinite presence of God, as in the garden of Eden, man was created by love; and only through love can he realize his full potential. All his different elements must find themselves, then amalgamate to produce total self-knowledge and an ultimate union. Tensions having been elim-inated, the two components of the being are suffused with calm, duality is transformed into unity, and all mental unrest is erased. The muscular and nervous contractions are liberated, and there at last are the green pastures promised by the Lord as a resting place.

This 'wedding' of mind and body can be attained initially by a complete state of relaxation in the stretched-out posture. Subsequently it may be reached seated, in a position of prayer, then during the series of postures that deal more fully with cementing the mind-body relationship. Each stage supports the following stage, and the collaboration is ultimately achieved.

Man is as the vault of a cathedral, where the name of God is pro-claimed, the echoes reverberating in every corner of the structure. The prayers in this series are man-made, like the echoes of God's name, resounding in the cathedral.

Only by being in constant pursuit of a state of unity can man attain it, and he must constantly overcome all the pitfalls of everyday life in the course of this pursuit. All the hallmarks of duality must be eliminated. Where these signs appear, the integration must again be undertaken, for the unison of mind-body demands mutual fidelity, not fidelity to those false 'household–gods' of interior friction, covetousness and obsessions, which must be destroyed. Then mind and body can feed and water themselves at the waters of repose, so that the soul itself may be nourished and renewed.

9. Yoga and chastity

Taking into consideration the fact that hatha yoga reinvigorates the natu-ral functions of the body, and that sexuality is one of those natural functions, it is probable that at the outset the discipline may actually increase sexual energy. Sexuality was given to each human being for the purpose of procreation, which is the execution of the divine work. But there is no doubt that an awareness of the body, the relaxation which gives birth to prayer, and the unison of mind and body will give the disciple the ability to approach the area of sexuality with more discern-ment. It will free him from all unhealthy ideas and procure him a more balanced existence. Sexuality is a natural instinct which will hardly be controlled or eradicated by force, shame, or a reluctance to acknowledge its presence. Lucidity, a clear understanding of the ultimate aspirations, and the ability to chose those aspirations, are much more likely to bring about a state of chastity.

All too often a need for affection is confused with sexual needs. Here once again mind and body should be linked, for if they are at variance, a desire for tenderness and affection is mistakenly interpreted by the body as sexual desire. This is frequently the reason for excessive sexuality.

All life was created by love – mankind; plants; animals. Without love, there is no Life, therefore man needs love. It should be given freely, openly, and unconditionally. Most human dramas are caused by egotism, covetousness, and possessiveness all masquerading as love, together with a general inability to define or identify love itself. And all this when love is so desperately needed and sought by all! Each individual should both give and accept affection with equal freedom and generosity, but how many are capable of this?

Most parents and grandparents are moved by some inner force to provide children with an abundance of disinterested love. They seem almost to form a ladder of communication between earth and heaven, which the children blithely climb. How much more difficult it is to pray to a celestial Father, when one has received nothing from an earthly father! The current violence of world youth must surely be the simple reaction of youth unloved.

Man has long cherished the desire to liberate himself from all physical attachments in order to consecrate his life entirely to God, and in spite of the personal difficulties and hardships that this dedication entails. But such aspirations are the privilege of a creature made in the image of God, his Creator. While vegetables and animals perpetuate themselves wholly spontaneously, man himself feels free to choose. This liberty leads to a number of sexual problems, as it is constantly abused and misused in ways which are universally apparent.

A number of 'God's fools' have found that in liberating themselves from carnal unions, they have been able to achieve a more intense consummation of the divine union, thus renewing life at its original source. This is no smothering of the sexual instinct by means of brute force, but by the sublimation of sexuality, which gives place to a relationship of pure and divine love between man and God.

It is in this sense that hatha yoga, with the help of divine grace, will effect a union with God, and help the Christian who has chosen chastity. It will show him the path to a better way of life by showing him the true face of love, and permitting him to be more aware, more available, and more conscious of his real needs. The postures will help him learn to accept his weaknesses and imperfections, and prevent his mind from wandering and dwelling upon unhealthy topics. The body is controlled by the mind, so the body reacts to any mental obsessions in kind. Relaxation and respiration persuade these obsessions to disperse, and the result is a complete realization of the total being. Immobility gives the ability to avoid all stimulating muscular contraction. Divine tenderness will be perceived, so that transparency will be experienced, and finally an unparalleled feeling of interior well-being. The wretched frustrations and worries of poor humanity have small value in the face of such joyous serenity.*

*Precise information about traditional yoga, the whole point of which is union with God, cannot be included here, as it is a very specialized field. In classical yoga sexual energy is transformed into spiritual energy by extremely complicated techniques.

42

Yoga will add another dimension to the relationship between husband and wife. The silences and immobile relaxation, without which all muscular stimulation is exhausting, will be shared so that the couple will ruly become 'one flesh'. During these flowing exchanges of joyful surrender, an inexpressible harmony is born. It is free from all covetousness, possessiveness, passion, and sensuality. The link which has been established between the couple is more powerful than the sexual union, for sex does not create this precious mutual participation which produces peace and concord. Fortunately, more often than not, most couples do experience this 'togetherness', which is quite removed from sensuality.

In order to share such experiences it is not necessary either to cheat or oppose nature. On the contrary, an awareness of, and obedience to nature are the keys to interior well-being and a climate where trust and intense tenderness can flourish.

The complementary polarities of two bodies, one masculine, the other feminine, are so balanced in each partner that the mutual surrender of the couple brings accord, rather than the discord so often produced by individual personal prejudice. The relaxed bodies of the man and the woman, lying together, evoke the 'profound sleep' into which God made man fall (Gen. 2, 25). This is truly one flesh, according to the will of him who created man. Carnal union gains a blossoming spiritual dimension in affirmation of the vocation of mankind as children of God, fashioned in his image.

Breathing

Yoga respiration is effected exclusively through the nose, which is specially equipped to filter the impurities in the air. The internal nasal passage forms a kind of keyboard comprising a number of notes, each of which has an individual function. Yoga respiration has a beneficial effect upon this keyboard, bringing it supplementary oxygenization and pranic energy. Pranic energy is a vital energy found in the air, together with all the chemical components. By means of a conscious movement, the nostrils are able to augment the system with this regenerating energy; the concentrated thought of man possesses the faculty to obtain and direct this source.

1. Conscious Breathing

(a) The processes of breathing

Conscious breathing is best effected while stretched out on the ground. Complete relaxation is the first necessity for each exercise; otherwise the exercises are of no benefit whatsoever. The face should always wear an expression of serenity, never a frown. No force should be employed; at first, simply observe and feel the natural functions. Begin by following the path of the air through the body, focus the attention on the sides of the nostrils, feeling the penetration of the air, the descent into the back of the throat, and the movement directly towards the lungs. Feel the warmth of the expulsion of the air, pinching both lips and nostrils lightly to expel all the air completely, but gently.

(b) Inhalation and exhalation

Eventually, these two very distinct phases should be fully observed and understood. Give particular attention to exhalation, as it empties the lungs. Also, it is of special interest to a western Christian, as it is synonymous with renunciation constantly renewed – the life of Christ constantly growing within man. From the physiological point of view, exhalation entirely relaxes the body. Slow exhalation produces a light internal effect which calms the mind. At first, allow the breath to come and go consciously and naturally, making sure that all tensions are released, so there is often the tendency to frown. While the Oriental must learn to inhale, the Westerner, too attached to his problems, must devote his attention to exhalation, which carries a physical and mental purification. This is a phase of abandon, of laying bare. Each intake of breath descends to the source of the profound being, to create a stripping and a rebirth. The relaxation of the believer leads to a recovery of the repose promised by God, and in the exhalation phase, conscious respiration corresponds to a voluntary death accepted by an old man who, during the following inhalation, is reborn as a new and better person. Here the image is one of waves, which recede and reform unceasingly.

This breath, drawn from the cosmos, unites mankind. Obedient to the rhythm of flux and influx, he is at one with the universe. Breathing is reintegration with the universal rhythm; man breathes with God, and with the whole of his creation. Little by little, all the irritations which provoke unnatural and unrhythmic movements are banished. Take notice of the ebb and flow of the air – when it penetrates, it is fresh, when it is rejected it is tepid, because it is charged with mental and physical impurities.

(c) Unblocking the diaphragm

Before embarking upon the great adventure of breathing, it is essential to bring mobility to the diaphragm. Modern life does not promote suppleness; fear, anguish, noise, and emotions of all sorts (as well as a sedentary life) are all obstacles to the proper functioning of the muscles.

The three following exercises should make a great deal of difference to stiff muscles:

(d) Rocking the pelvis

Stand upright, placing one hand flat above the navel, and the other on the back, above the kidneys. Contract the muscles of the buttocks, then release them. Gradually, become more and more aware of the articulation in this area, and of the rocking of the pelvis. Because of the intermediary action of this articulation, there will be no blockage of the diaphragm.

(e) The four paws (A 4 and 5)

Propped up on the hands, arms and knees stretched straight out, breathe out, curving the back. Breathe in, arching the kidneys. Breathing out again, lift the head to look at the navel. Rock several times, being conscious of the results of the movements in the stomach region. The diaphragm moves, rallying the internal organs for the exhalation, while the inhalation causes the thoracic cage to leave the lungs free.

(f) The half-bridge (F 15)

To reinforce the benefits of the preceding exercise:

Stretch out on the back, then with the help of the hands, lift up the pelvis, so the body is supported by the soles of the feet, the elbows, and the nape of the neck. In this position, breathe deeply, allowing the stomach to inflate. As a result, the diaphragm will become much suppler. If there should be any feeling of tiredness, loosen the posture; sliding gently, stretch out the arms behind the head, stretch, then exhale, to begin the unwinding of the spinal column, one vertebra after the other. Throughout, be conscious of the mobility of the column. Inhale, then descend the vertebrae on the following exhalation, making sure that the lumbar region is absolutely flat in front of the muscles of the buttocks. This will ensure that at the conclusion of the exercise the spinal column will lie more evenly and completely flat on the ground. This progressive stretching and unwinding on an exhalation provides an excellent massage, soothing the central nervous system, which is concerned with each side of the vertebral column.

This exercise is extremely soothing, and may be practised before a relaxation, as it is a good preparatory exercise.

2. Complete yoga respiration

Complete yoga respiration is composed of the three following stages: abdominal, thoracic, and clavicular.

Abdominal respiration is totally neglected by current respiratory programmes. Certain professors of gymnastics encourage absolute firmness in this region, which of course produce stiffness in the shoulders. In yoga, inhalation and exhalation cover three stages, so that the air cells of the lungs are multiplied and regenerated. Breathing takes six directions – above, below, in front, at the back, at the sides.

Exercises in the three respiratory stages are begun by lying stretched out on the ground.

(a) The three respiratory stages

1. Place the hands end to end at the level of the navel, following the movement of the stomach as it inflates and deflates. Do nothing; simply observe, without interfering.
2. Raise the hands to each side of the thoracic region, similarly observing the enlargement and reduction provoked by the respiration.
3. Place the hands on the clavicular region, also observing the effect of the respiration.

Afterwards, observe the movement in the totality of the three stages by placing one hand on the abdomen and the other on the thoracic area. Stay relaxed at all times – never force anything. Allow the natural respiratory processes to take their course unhindered.

(b) Respiration through the back

Swing over on to the stomach, being aware of the breathing in the position, and feeling the pressure on the abdomen. Make a chandelier with the hands, elbows at the height of the shoulders, then with undivided attention, follow the course of the respiration without attempting to modify it. The pressure upon the abdomen obliges the back to raise itself, giving access to the pulmonary regions, which are rarely throroughly oxygenated. Notice the hardening of the abdomen, as this provides a solid basis for the postures on the flat of the stomach, such as the cobra, bow, grasshopper, and so on. For a Christian, the posture on the flat of the stomach and respiration in that position both have relevance to .prayer, and are very frequently used in that context. They represent man showing humility, and surrendering to the earth which supports him. Observation ceases of its own accord, the mind is soothed, the back is entirely relaxed, and all gives place to prayer.

It is possible to intensify respiration through the back by exhaling from a greater depth. The diaphragm, being against the ground, is blocked, so that the breath is exhaled through the back. The result is an appreciable increase in the air cells of the lungs.

3. Respiratory rhythms

In order to discover the respiratory rhythms, first return to the position on the back. In the same way that in music certain notes are held longer than others, in respiration the phases may be prolonged or shortened. These phases are: intake of breath; retention of breath in the full lungs; expulsion of breath, and retention of the empty lungs.

As the whole point of this work is the attainment of a mental calm conducive to prayer, the programme is exclusively confined to simple, natural, respiratory rhythms. The respiratory rhythm is a kind of magic key which opens the door to a calm and serene interior. The regularity of the breathing virtually provides an internal spring–clean which neutralizes mental irritants and regularizes the energies of the physical body; this leads eventually to sound and restorative sleep. Conscious respiration regularly sweeps out the mental and physical structures leaving only peace, a climate in which meditation and prayer will flourish. The eyes close naturally, while the mind threads itself into the sound of the respiration. The mind should not stir from this position, then contact will be established with the whole of creation. Again, grace and prayer are created quite spontaneously. Could any Christian remain insensible to this divinely given rhythm of life which is absorbed with each inhalation, bringing the kind of nourishment upon which man originally based his existence? No, he will live each breath like the first breath breathed by the Love of God. This is the soothing breath which brings total peace as it penetrates all parts of the body; the divine hand which fashioned the first man continues to give life.

Lie stretched out on the back. Place one hand on the abdomen, the other on the thoracic region. Exhale, being as conscious of the process as though it were a completely new experience. Inhale spontaneously, simultaneously threading the mind into the light noise made by the air as it passes through the throat. Then gradually feel the regularisation of the breath. Now begin with a very simple rhythm:

abdominal inhalation	once	
thoracic ,,	,,	3 times
clavicular ,,	,,	
retention; lungs full	once	once
abdominal exhalation	,,	
thoracic exhalation	,,	3 times
clavicular exhalation	,,	
retention; lungs empty	,,	once

During the following yoga programme, this rhythm may be modified – 3/1/3/1 to 3/2/5/2, a simple classical rhythm.

The precise meaning of 'once' differs according to the individual; rules should be devised and guided by temperament. But fatigue promotes tension, so that it would be quite pointless to prolong any exercise to the point of strain or exhaustion. Never change the rhythm during the course of a single session. Try to breathe as subtly as possible, because the words 'profound respiration' imply a minimum length of breath. In making a breath shorter, respiration becomes more thorough and efficient. To control the length of breath, place a warm palm in front of the nose.

A number of respiratory rhythms exist which prolong one of the four aforementioned phases. This is because the use of these rhythms by the yogis of India and Tibet become positive exploits. They are able to raise or reduce their temperature because the body has been brought to such a state of alertness that the perceptions are heightened, and in consequence desired reactions may be produced.

Limit the exhalation to double that of the inhalation. Never on any account try to exceed this, particularly during the long retentions of the full or empty lungs. It cannot be stressed strongly enough that the surveillance of a qualified master is as essential as a body which is free from all tension. This work suggests that the body be used as a spring-board to prayer and availability to God, so it is more relevant to limit the programme to simple rhythms. The more complicated rhythms have quite a different objective, in that they induce an excessive mobility of the mind. Regular respiration works naturally and spontaneously to replace man in the soothing rhythm of nature.

Subsequently it will be found possible to practise alternative respiration, which balances the positive and negative energies in the body, and could be used as a preparation for prayer.

Plug first the left then the right nostril with a finger, breathing in through the unblocked nostril. Hold the breath for an instant, then exhale through the other nostril. Slow down the breath as much as possible, then to return it more deeply, shorten the length of the breath, returning it as subtly as possible. The free fingers should feel the sensation.

For this exercise, a comfortable seat is needed. The spinal column should be held straight, but not rigid, while the face should be decontracted in order to facilitate the circulation of energy, otherwise there may be adverse effects rather than beneficial ones.

Do not change the rhythms during a single session of exercises.

In order to find the correct rhythm so that no tensions will be provoked either in the face or the body, allow the breath to come and go as it will; the intelligence of the body should take over. If there is the slightest sign of fatigue, relax.

During relaxations, the breath will relax the body and lead it into the postures for which so many preparations are being made.

F. The Do-In, or warm-up

The Do-In is the last set before the postures. Pay careful attention to the suppleness of all the articulations of the body, especially those of the hands and feet. A number of energies course through the body, and upon this concept is based the principle of acupuncture. In practical yoga, the Do-In may be defined as digital acupuncture. Important meridians divide the hands; these are the meridians of the lungs, the large intestine, sexual energy, triple warm-up, the heart, and the small intestine. The feet are crossed by the meridians of the liver, the spleen, the stomach, the bladder, the gall-bladder, and the kidneys. Any action upon any specific meridian requires long and minute study, but the wisdom of nature, always being ready and well-equipped for action, distributes and dispenses this energy of its own volition, and can be relied upon to do so intelligently and promptly – just as long as the body is supple and free from all tension. The Do-In exercises are very simple, and within the scope of all and sundry.

Manipulate, stretch, bend and turn each finger of both hands, and each toe of both feet. Manipulate the wrists and the ankles, in order to mass the palms of the hands and the soles of the feet. Tap the arms and legs lightly. Neck, and nape of the neck exercises act upon the meridians equally well in preparation for the postures. Twisting is important, as it acts upon the meridian of the centre, and it is here that significant activity, slowed down by a sedentary life, takes place. Pat the chest and the back, then try some vowel sounds on an exhalation. The human body is a receiver which collects colours, sounds and smells, and in the Do-In these are called Ki energy. The body collects this energy through pressure points which are situated under the skin in proximity to the meridians, which transport the energy to the whole body. In a completely healthy body Ki energy circulates freely, but the individual who is tired or ill will find that Ki energy is not circulating, and that the arms and feet are tender to the touch. It is therefore necessary to disperse the energy by means of massage, manipulation, and the suppling of the articulations. Hatha yoga postures carry this out: one of the reasons why the discipline protects the health of those who practise it. At the spiritual level, with which this work is mainly concerned, the Do-In and the hatha yoga postures permeate the body, bestowing upon the owner the power and desire for spontaneous prayer, and making him aware of God's divine presence and receptive to his word.

G. Sitting-on-the-ground

This is a key posture in yoga and prayer. There are many variants, all demanding suppleness in the articulation of the hips, the knees, and the feet, and requiring a general relaxation of the muscles. Perseverance and patience are often necessary, but some very stiff pupils have often managed to hold one of the sitting postures very comfortably after only a few month's training. The following preparatory exercises are necessary:

1. Sit down on the ground, legs stretched out in front. After having

tolled the legs, bend one, catching the foot with both hands. Manipulate the toes with the hands, straightening then bending them. Manipulate the soles of the feet, then tap them. Catch the right foot in the right hand and make the articulations of the leg function by stretching the leg, then bringing it under the back of the knee.

2. Begin again on the other side. Bend one of the legs. Place the heel as near as possible to the buttock of the same side. Place the hands on the knees, or on the sides, taking care that the back is straight, but not rigid. Breathe calmly; change to the other leg. Then try the exercise with both legs bent together on each side. At first, it will be easier if a small cushion is placed at the small of the back (J38–39).

3. Bring both feet under the buttocks, taking the bamboo posture. Sit on the heels, toes folded. The hands lie on the thighs, the chest is held lightly back, chin agains the sternum. Breathe calmly and deeply (J40).

4. Sit on the ground, the legs forming a V. Place the hands behind, in order to straighten the back. Bring the right leg to lodge inside the left at the height of the thighs. If the bent knee does not touch the ground, do not force it. Without forcing, decontract, loosen, and breathe calmly; this is the correct weight at which the knees should descend. Alternate (J41).

5. With the aid of the hands, bring up the feet so that the soles are facing the back as far as possible. Supple the articulation of the ankles by manipulating the feet with the hands. No brute force should be employed. Bring the head down to touch the soles of the feet.

6. If there should be any difficulty in holding the sitting position correctly, use the wall as a prop. With legs V-shaped, wedge the posterior against the wall, and re-erect the back. Place first one leg then the other to sit tailor-fashion, in a perfect posture – that is, one foot behind the other, or if possible, in a lotus; legs locked together, the soles of the feet turned towards the sky. The main consideration must always be – no forcing. If it should be necessary, do not hesitate to use the wall during the initial stages. Preferably, raise the posterior placing the knees easily on the ground, so that before concluding, the simple sitting position may be taken correctly and with the right balance. The back should be straight, but not rigid; this is done by raising the arms above the head, palm pressed to palm, then bringing the wrists to the top of the head. The back having been re-erected, bring the arms down without modifying the position of the back.

7. The Carmelite posture supples the ankles and the articulations of the knees. If there is any stiffness, a small bench may be used. The measurements are given here.

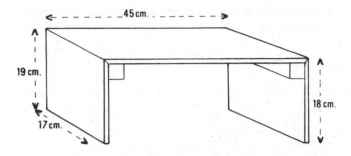

H. Awareness of the body

Awareness of the body is the last stage before the postures. It is easier to be aware of the body when it is moving, but for the awareness during mobile postures, some preparation is necessary.

This exercise is of particular importance and interest in yoga and prayer, because of all sacred gestures – gestures made in relation to prayer. These gestures offer to God everything contained in the depth of the soul. So how can they be automatic, like those of a robot?

A priest who celebrates Mass with conscious gestures, pouring out his profound being, communicates the intensity of his personal prayer to his acolytes and his congregation. It is impossible to live according to the precepts of hatha yoga without this 'living presence'. It is impossible to pray if the accompanying gestures are superficial and automatic. This is one of the number of aspects of yoga discipline which facilitate prayer at a profound and intense level, thereby granting the child an authentic vision of the Father.

Current life-styles are exhausting because they dissociate all elsewhere. Where there is conscious presence, there is no fatigue. Where great physical effort is involved, the instinct is to reassemble all available forces, and for an instant, mental gymnastics are discontinued. In hatha yoga, as in prayer, dancing, and all the sacred rites, it is essential that all levels should be reunited, so that all gestures and attitudes will be sincere.

One example is the posture of resurrection, which is a balanced upright position. Loosen the shoulders, relax the muscles of the back, centre the weight low in the body, then begin to walk very slowly, feeling every movement of the body. Bend the knees, then straighten them; hold the pose. Feel how the ground articulates the feet; mass the soles thoroughly; never walk on stiff feet; remain supple. Feel the articulation of the hips and the balancing movements of the arms, at the same time being aware that the feet lift, falling first on the right then on the left. Allow the breath to exhale from the area of the navel, while poised on one foot. Lift the other foot on an inhalation; be present. This conscious attitude brings total availability, so that prayer may follow this simple exercise.

Follow in the footsteps of the Lord, placing the feet carefully, attentively, and lovingly, as though to be indelibly marked by the imprint of the divine footprints.

Into your steps I will put my steps, Lord,
For they are the source of Life.
Into your steps will I place mine, Lord,
For they are the source of joy.
Life and joy flow from your steps, Lord,
And I will follow you for all Eternity.
Others will follow in my steps, Lord,
We shall greet each other, and unite,
Fitting our steps into your steps, Lord,
Forming a circle of joy and eternal life.

Now enter into yoga and prayer, and the body will become a living temple in the image of God.

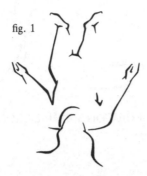

fig. 1

1. RELAXATION ON THE BACK

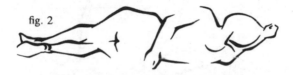

fig. 2

2. RELAXATION ON THE SIDE: POSTURE OF A SLEEPING CHILD

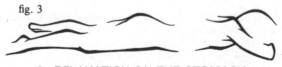

fig. 3

3. RELAXATION ON THE STOMACH

1, 2 and 3. Stop all muscular and mental activity. Relax both body and mind. Abandon the muscles to the law of gravity, to procure deeper relaxation. Be aware of the breath; feeling the natural 'come-and-go', listen to the slight noise made by the respiration in the back of the throat. The body is now completely relaxed.

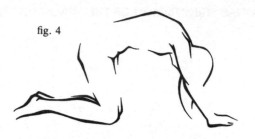

fig. 4

4. PURIFYING EXHALATION

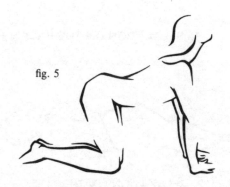

fig. 5

5. SPONTANEOUS INHALATION

4 and 5. UNBLOCKING THE DIAPHRAGM

4 and 5. Restore the natural function of the diaphragm. Exhale (4) in order to get rid of the stale air. Allow the inhalation to be made spontaneously. (5) Vary the following exercise by manoeuvring a bent leg so that the knee moves in the direction of the chin. Return the leg on the inhalation.

Series B: STRETCHING, MUSCULAR WARM-UPS, RECONSTRUCTION OF THE BACK

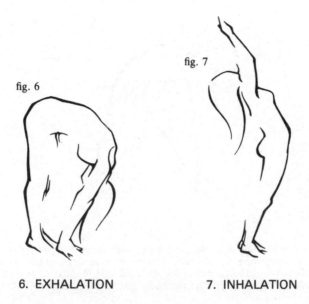

fig. 7

fig. 6

6. EXHALATION   7. INHALATION

6 and 7. STRETCHING AND WARM–UPS

SLOW MASSAGE OF THE SPINAL CORD, gentle stretching of the vertebrae on an exhalation, for the reinvigoration of the nervous system. In 7., the back is reconstructed on an inhalation. Straighten up again slowly, so that the vertebrae can replace themselves one on top of the other, like coins. This exercise is a preparation for the greeting of the sun, and should be practised as a greeting. Exhalation is purifying, inhalation invigorating.

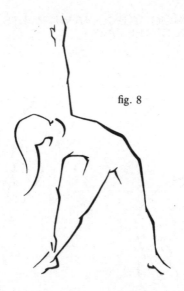

fig. 8

8.

THE TRIANGLE: aeration of the lungs in their costal region. On an inhalation, cross the arms, lowering them on either side. Having filled the lungs, exhale. Thoroughly air the lungs by breathing through the stretched side. Repeat on the other side. This aeration of the lungs purifies the body, and is of special benefit after 'flu, or colds.

Series C: POSTURES ON THE KNEES

The hands may be placed in different positions – at the sides, crossed, behind the back (arms held, or palm against palm, as in prayer) or in front, arms held so that the vertebral column is stretched. Or, sit cross-legged, knees touching the ground on each side, so that the column is not off-balance. The main object is to supple the spinal column, but without any kind of rough handling, so that it is prepared for more complicated movements. Also, all the different arm positions give the lungs a chance to air themselves thoroughly.

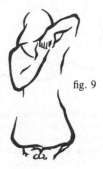

fig. 9

9. OPENING THE THORACIC CAGE

Posture 9 represents the maximum opening of the thoracic cage, preparing the pupil for much deeper breathing. While upright, breathe in. While lowering the forehead to touch the ground, breathe out. Repeat on the other side.

Series D: PREPARATION ON THE BACK

Well-toned stomach-muscles keep the back straight, so that the diaphragm is able to massage the viscera and the plexus. Respiration is also improved.

fig. 10

10. THE WORK OF THE ABDOMINALS

The body is on the ground, quite relaxed. Breathing in, raise both head and legs a little. As the knees straighten and stretch, observe the feet. The small of the back should not be curved; regulate the raising of the head and legs so that the small of the back is absolutely flat, otherwise there is a risk that the vertebral discs may be damaged. There are a number of exercises which will tone the stomach muscles, other than the one illustrated, and some will be found in a later section. Exercise 10 has the advantage of aiding the relaxation of the muscles on exhaling, when the posture is dropped.

Series E: CLOSED POSTURES. BEGIN ON THE BACK

Now begin to work the spinal column more thoroughly. Before practising the whole series of postures, gradually make the body more flexible.

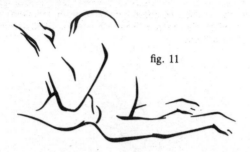

fig. 11

11.

THE FOETUS: a soothing closed posture. Separate the bent legs on the ground, so that the small of the back is not damaged. Slowly lift hands and feet, then, hug the knees with the arms, and breathe calmly through the back. This is a posture of surrender and trust, where renewal is effected by the great universal matrix.

This posture is helpful in cases of back trouble.

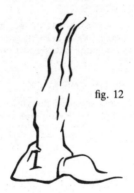

fig. 12

12.

THE CANDLE: a reverse soothing posture. If the arms are raised to the height of the chest, it may also be a posture of equilibrium. It is said that the body does not age when it is thus reversed, as when the circulation of the blood and the lymphatic system are reversed, the legs and all the organs are provisionally lightened. The diaphragm is activated in such a way that those suffering from asthma are likely to obtain some relief. The stretching of the cervical vertebrae and the glottal humming both calm the mind, while the body experiences a sensation of insubstantiality. This is because of the unusual use of the force of gravity, the soles of the feet being exposed to a positive solar energy, instead of a negative terrestrial energy. To take the posture, lie stretched out on the ground. Bend the knees, without curving the small of the back, then, aided first by the hands then by the elbows, raise the legs on an inhalation. The legs are slack, the feet are not pointed, there is no tension. To come down, bend the legs, and place the feet on the ground gently, without banging down the heels. If there is any difficulty in raising the body, do not worry, simply keep the legs in the air, straight, but not rigid, with the body on the ground. Just think of the complete posture, and after a time the result will be the actual accomplishment of the complete posture. For praying, the body is suffused by the warmth from the burning of the heart, as the body has been raised like a flame.

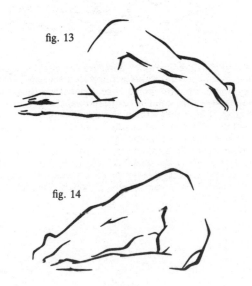

fig. 13

fig. 14

13 and 14

THE CHARIOT: a soothing closed reversed posture. The spinal column bends more, stretching the spinal cord, and the nervous system is invigorated. Do not force the feet to touch the ground, simply allow the weight of the legs to pull them down, so that they are utterly relaxed. Begin like a candle in the stretched out position, then bend the legs, keeping the feet flat. With the help of the arms, swing up the lower half of the body. These movements should be controlled from the interior, using the minimum number of muscles. The column is worked even more during the dynamic phase, which consists of two returns to the lengthwise position, with a swing back up again before becoming immobile. The body swings into the universal rhythm quite spontaneously, just as the flowers open and close in the heat of the sun. These are slow and harmonious gestures. In traditional yoga, the chariot permits the aeration and fertilisation of the earth, the posture permeating the body so that receptivity to cosmic vibrations is improved.

Series F: OPEN POSTURES: BEGIN ON THE BACK

The new flexibility of the vertebral column has increased the flexibility of other areas. Preparation having been made, work may now begin on the vertebrae, so that eventually they become completely supple.

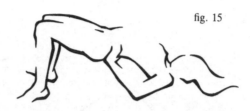

fig. 15

15.

THE HALF-BRIDGE is an exercise which will unblock the diaphragm. After more deep breathing, swing the arms behind the head, then descend slowly on an exhalation, placing the spinal column, from the nape of the neck to the coccyx, evenly on the ground. Stop the descent during inhalation, then continue on the following exhalation. While spreading the small of the back and the buttocks evenly on the ground, contract the abdomen. Then, slowly, one after the other, slide the legs a little along the ground, so that the spinal column is laid down as flat as a plank. This is one of the most difficult of the hatha yoga postures, so it should be perfected by degrees. All the practice periods will provide a complete massage for the back. It is a very soothing exercise, suitable for times when relaxation is difficult.

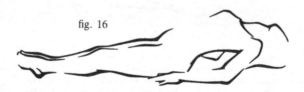

fig. 16

16.

THE FISH is a toning posture. Respiration takes place at the height of the lungs. Supported by the elbows, bend, and 'breathe' the chest open. In relation to prayer, this corresponds to an opening of the heart. To come down again, allow the head to slide without any adjustment, as there is a risk of damaging the cervical vertebrae. If the nape of the neck is very stiff, ease the position with a small cushion.

The complete posture is made in a lotus, and may eventually be tried cross-legged, then in a half-lotus.

fig. 17

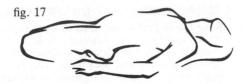

17.

THE DIAMOND, or great reversal, is a particularly toning open posture. The maximum opening of the chest which occurs is almost akin to a gift offering. The plexus is then able to perform a soothing function, and the stretching gives a kind of toning recharge. Everything must happen naturally, no force should be used. Cross the arms, placing them under the small of the back for support, or else raise the arms above the head, to give maximum stretch to the solar plexus. Breathe deeply and regularly, so that the recharging of the body is experienced internally. Do not try to adjust the position again, but allow the nape of the neck to slide across the ground, open out the legs one after the other, and lie on the back, completely relaxed.

fig. 18

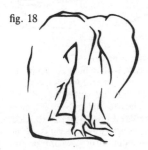

18.

THE HERO is an open, toning posture. Be sure that the weight of the body rests entirely on the knees. Initially, the hands may be placed in the curve of the buttocks. If the nerves of the nape of the neck are fragile, weave the fingers together to form a support for it. Gradually, the spinal column will become supple, so that finally, the hands may be placed on the ankles. Breathe deeply and regularly, in order to stretch the solar plexus; the arms should neither be linked nor supported. The open posture of the heart represents availability to God. Do not hold this posture for more than a few seconds, as there is a risk of inducing a fainting fit.

Series F (a set): OPEN POSTURES FLAT ON THE STOMACH

These postures support the rise and fall of the abdomen during respiration. They gradually effect a complete flexibility of the vertebral column, as the head, legs, body, or all simultaneously are raised. The work of the column is modified by the position of the open arms – at the sides; held straight out; bent. The open postures promote an intensity of activity in the endocrinal glands, the thyroid and adrenal glands being particularly affected. The liver is stretched, and the kidneys assembled and compressed. Those with over-active thyroids should take these postures with head lowered, chin agains the sternum, like those who have trouble with the nape of the neck.

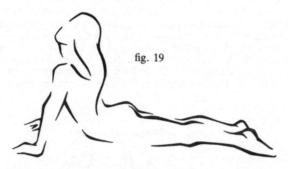

fig. 19

19.

THE COBRA is an open bracing posture.

THE SPHINX is an easier version with which to begin. First, keep the arms on the ground, stretched out from the shoulders. Support should be provided by the fingertips, not the elbows, so that the spinal column is fortified.

There are several approaches to the cobra. Beginners should set out by lying flat on the ground, arms stretched out from the shoulders. Rise gradually through successive exhalations, then, before any tension is felt in the shoulders, stop. Bring the bent arms down on an exhalation. Ascent on an inhalation. Repeat three times. Directly the arms bend, the chest may also be raised, the hands being under the shoulders. The hands should provide as little support as possible, so that the spinal column will work. The arm movements bend the vertebral column: arms folded at the back; palms together; hands crossed.

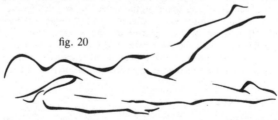

fig. 20

20.

THE HALF-GRASSHOPPER and the grasshopper are the open bracing postures which complete work in a different area of the vertebral column. In the half-grasshopper, the body is held steady while one leg is raised on an intake of breath, then lowered on an exhalation. The hands may be placed at the sides, arms bent.

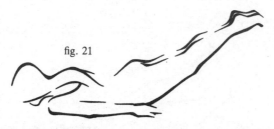

fig. 21

21.

THE GRASSHOPPER: support is taken by the hands, which are either held flat, or crossed under the thighs while the legs are raised. The nerves of the adrenal system are activated. Do not practise before bed time.

In both grasshopper postures, exhale while slowly lowering the legs.

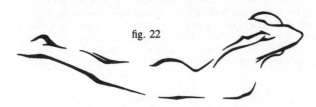

fig. 22

22.

THE ARCH is an open posture which aids the decontraction of the muscles of the abdomen. Inhale, first tightening, then loosening the abdomen. It would be equally bracing simply to hold the posture while breathing regularly.

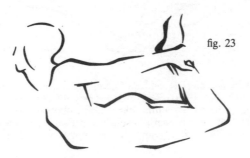

fig. 23

23.

THE BOW is an intensely bracing open posture. The arms are not linked, and remain completely relaxed now that the back has been thoroughly decontracted. The knees are placed apart, kept at the same level, then brought gently back, one against the other, so that the traction is equal on each side of the column.

The knees may also be kept on the ground without raising the torso, in which case, the posture is called THE CAMEL. At first, do not hold the breath, but continue to breath regularly. When the thoracic cage has been prepared, the lungs may be kept full of air for a moment, then gently released.

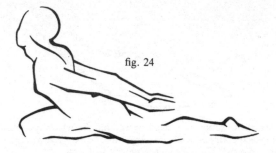

fig. 24

24.

THE DOVE: symbol of peace. This is a very beautiful and harmonious posture, where the body is rebuilt very slowly. Balancing on the lower part of the body, hold the arms out behind the back in order to open the chest. Chin thrust forward, breathe deeply and calmly. The abdomen receives a massage. The hands may also be placed one on top of the other on one knee, while the column readjusts itself. Or alternatively, raise the arms above the head, like a cover. This is a very lovely posture of prayer, evoking the spiritual aspirations of man, anchored to the ground.

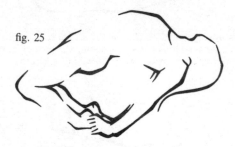

fig. 25

25.

THE REVERSE BOW is a special posture of equilibrium. Begin on the knees, hands flat down on each foot. Raise the knees, keeping the chin against the sternum. When the legs are raised, swing the head back and breathe regularly. This is a bracing posture, and when properly controlled, perfect for prayer. With reversed balance, the body offers both immobile and mobile symbols in the form of a wheel.

Series G: CLOSED POSTURES

After the open posture work has been begun, the body is closed by soothing postures. Those suffering from insomnia will find these preferable, as they give a soothing massage to the solar plexus, which then folds. The spinal column stretches the nerve endings, and this reinvigorates the nervous system.

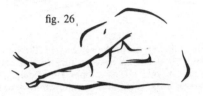

fig. 26

26.

THE PLIERS is a classic posture which possesses particularly soothing qualities. First, sit down, then swing the arms into the air on an inhalation. In articulating the seat at hip level, the trunk is propelled forward. Stay relaxed – do not use force. Make the movement three times very slowly on an inhalation. In exhaling before remaining mobile in the posture, stretching is facilitated very gradually and pleasantly. Initially, the posture may also be taken lying stretched out, arms taken back on an inhalation, returning towards the thighs on an exhalation. Then the head is lifted and the hands slide towards the feet, pulling the trunk.

An alternative is as follows: place crossed arms under the knees, trunk against the thighs, allowing the calves to slide slowly across the ground, but without losing the contact between trunk and thigh. Complete relaxation is essential.

The pliers evokes man's efforts to accomplish his mission.

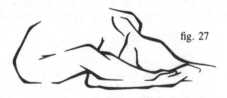

fig. 27

27.

THE STAR or THE OYSTER is a beautiful posture. It provokes maximum stretching of the spinal column at the level of the seat, and also a compression of the abdomen, which is accentuated by deep and regular respiration placed in the back. It aids the seat, the knees, and the feet, which are supported by the hands. It is a posture of humility and surrender, particularly if the forehead is laid on the feet. Loosen up well, without forcing any movement at any time. Bring down the head gradually, and at the same rate as the exhalations; this should be done easily and naturally. Although this is a soothing posture, within a certain closed circuit, it is also invigorating.

With the soles of the feet, then the hands, slowly turning towards the sky, energy is able to circulate through the body without escaping.

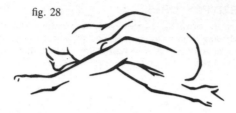

fig. 28

28.

THE TORTOISE symbolizes the retreat of the senses. It is the sign of new beginnings, and extremely soothing. It is not an easy posture to take, and to start with, it should be controlled only on one side at a time. The abdomen being compressed, stretch the upper portion of the torso and breathe calmly into the posture.

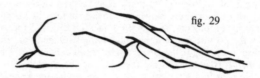

fig. 29

29.

MUSLIM PRAYER. This natural stretching of the spinal column is best carried out after all the work of the vertebral column, and above all after the open postures in series F.

Take this very easily at first: bend over to the stomach, lie flat on the stomach; now take the sitting position on the heels, then the upright position. This begins to replace the vertebrae, a process which is completed by the following posture.

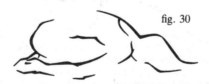

fig. 30

30.

THE BENT LEAF or POSTURE OF ELIJAH: a posture of vertebral and mental repose, which is described in detail in the text. None of the bending postures should be undertaken lightly, or without proper instruction. These postures very gently completely rebuild the back on an inhalation, the arms being held open in an expansive gesture of welcome.

Series H: THE TORSIONS or TWISTING POSTURES

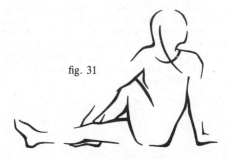

fig. 31

31.

SITTING TORSION is bracing. At first, simply bend a leg, bringing the right foot back against the internal part of the left knee, which should be flat on the ground. Supporting the buttocks with the right hand, turn slowly on an exhalation. When the maximum torsion has been achieved, hold the position, stay quite relaxed, and breathe calmly. Return slowly on a long exhalation. Before twisting the body in the opposite direction, lift the arms up into the air, crossing the hands. This will replace the vertebrae. The torsion may be embellished by the movement shown in Fig. 31 – the right foot is placed on the exterior of the left knee, then the left leg, which is on the ground, is bent. This torsion is partly the lotus, and partly the half-lotus if the right arm is placed behind the waist and the right foot is caught and placed at the height of the left thigh. Repeat on the other side. This torsion fortifies the kidneys; God probes the kidneys and the heart.

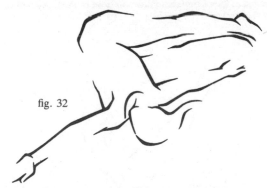

fig. 32

32.

RECUMBENT TORSION is reinvigorating as well as soothing, and most suitable for beginners. Stretch out on the ground, then on an inhalation, raise bent legs, as though sitting on an imaginary chair. On an exhalation bring the knees down on the left side, turning the head to the right. Stretch the legs gently to lengthen them, remaining relaxed during a few minutes of calm breathing. To return, bend the legs, bring them towards the face, then put the feet on the ground, allowing the legs to slide out straight. Repeat on the other side.

Series I: POSTURES OF EQUILIBRIUM – BALANCE AND CO-ORDINATION

There are a number of these postures, but this series will confine itself to the simplest. Their advantages have already been enumerated elsewhere in the text, but it cannot be stated too often that they provide a renewal, or reflowering.

Remain completely relaxed, like a supple blade of grass well rooted in the earth. Make sure that neither the ankles nor the face are clenched. The eyes should be focused on a specific point, but without any contraction. Breathe calmly and regularly through the hara, above the navel.

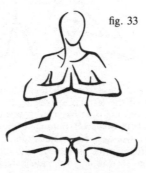

fig. 33

33.

THE FROG: this is one of the easiest postures. The legs should always be wide apart, with the buttocks resting on the heels, which are close together. In order to maintain balance, the arms are crossed. Hands joined, raise the arms above the head, re-set the back, then bring them down in front of the chest without modifying the position of the back.

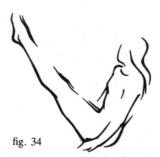

fig. 34

34.

THE BOAT: while taking this posture, be careful not to damage the lumbar region. The body should be aerial, held up at each side by the fingertips. This posture leads into the pliers posture: catch the feet with the hands and raise them in the air. The pliers is very bracing, and should not be overdone.

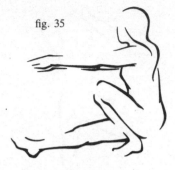

fig. 35

35.

THE EAGLE: the foot stretched out in front, so that it can be placed on the ground, or raised up high. The important thing is to find the correct balance.

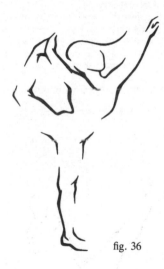

fig. 36

36.

THE GAZELLE or DANCER is an almost aerial posture of equilibrium. The supporting ankle must remain supple, respiration should be calm and regular, the gaze held steady and quite still, and the face relaxed.

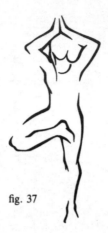

fig. 37

37.

THE TREE is the great classic of all the postures of equilibrium, and it may be executed in a number of different ways.

Lift the foot, lodging it against the opposite inside thigh, or well hooked up, as in the half-lotus. For balancing purposes, cross the arms, then lift them above the head, palm to palm, and stretch the vertebral column on an inhalation. On an exhalation, bring the hands up above the head, opening them in a cutting movement, then bring them down towards the chest, joining them in prayer. Breathe calmly and regularly.

The tree is a symbol of solidity for the Christian, representing his establishment in the faith.

Series J: SITTING POSTURES

Figs. 38–46 are complementary to the text in the preparation for these postures, and they are quite easy to follow. The attainment of the lotus is not of primary importance – on the contrary, the first essential is a good 'seat'! It is important that a cushion be used, so that the knees can stay on the ground without any difficulty. The knees and the navel should create a triangle. The feet are placed one in front of the other, the position being given stability by the absolute control with which the posture is constructed. Never force the knees; they should be brought down to the ground by their own weight, because of the relaxation of the leg muscles. The cushion should be used to raise the seat.

The half-pliers in Fig. 42 is taken by placing the feet on the interior of the opposite thigh, or at the height of the thigh. The arms are raised on an inhalation, while on an exhalation, the hands slide along the stretched out leg. This posture stretches the muscles at the back of the thighs, which are shortened by a sedentary life.

To avoid any vertebral damage, only elementary instruction is given here. As no instruction on postural technique is included, those who require further information should consult specialist literature on the subject.

During the postures, all breathing should be calm and regular. The breath may be held lightly, but more complicated respiratory techniques should be practised only under the surveillance of a qualified person. Holding the breath makes the body very alert, and possibly too impetuous!

All the illustrated postures do not constitute a complete sequence. The body should be prepared for the postures by the simple exercises which have been described here. The open bracing postures require about nineteen hours preparation, then activity should be limited to the closed postures, in order to prepare for a good night's refreshing sleep.

BEGINNING STAGE: A1–15; B6–7; C9; D10; E11; F15, 16, 19 (only in the sphinx) F20, 24; G26, 29, 30; H32, I35.

After a few weeks introduce the following: B8; E12; F17 (one leg bent at the side, the other stretched out) F19 in the cobra; F21, 22; G27; H31; I37; J42 (foot inside the opposite thigh.)

Other more complicated postures may be attempted later. If time is limited, it is better to perfect a small number of postures, than to scamp a large number. The right attitude may be established at the outset by pausing for a moment of quiet calm, so that all physical and mental activities may be left behind. Exhale deeply, inhale spontaneously, stretching the back. In the mornings, take an open bracing posture, then a simple closed posture. In the evening, do a candle, a chariot, a classical pliers, or one of the variants, a balancing posture.

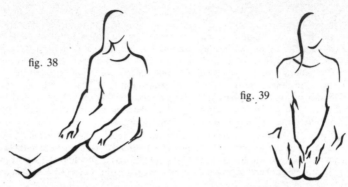

fig. 38

fig. 39

38. & 39. PREPARATION FOR THE SITTING POSTURE

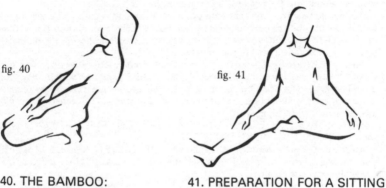

fig. 40

fig. 41

**40. THE BAMBOO:
HELPS THE FEET**

**41. PREPARATION FOR A SITTING
POSTURE**

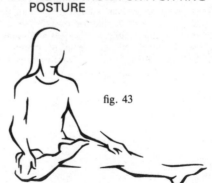

fig. 42

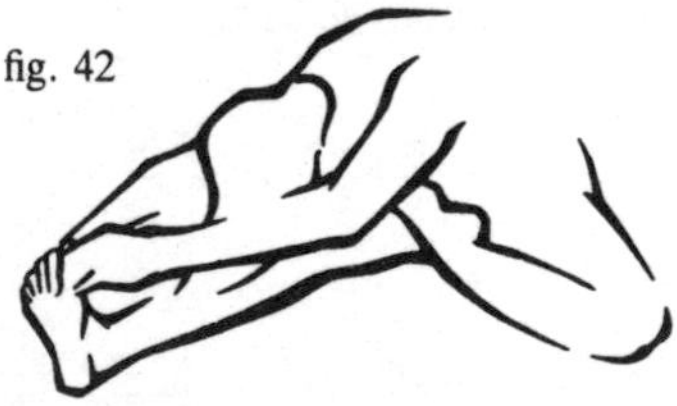

fig. 43

**42. THE HALF-PLIERS:
CLOSED POSTURE PREPARING
FOR A SITTING POSTURE**

**43. PREPARATION FOR THE
LOTUS**

44. THE LOTUS

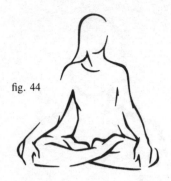

fig. 44

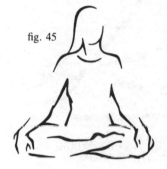

fig. 45

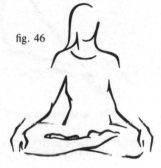

fig. 46

45. & 46. SIMPLIFIED VARIANTS OF THE LOTUS

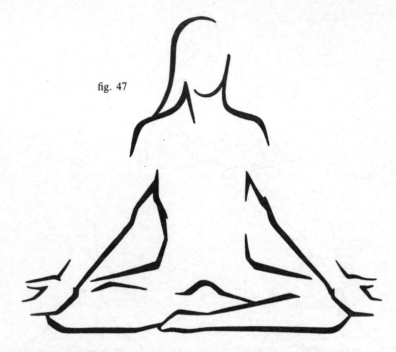

fig. 47

**47. VERY STABLE SITTING POSTURE – USE A VERY THICK
CUSHION SO THAT THE KNEES STAY ON THE GROUND**

III BODY SYMBOLISM IN PRAYER

A. The posture of Elijah or the bent leaf posture
'And Elijah went up to the top of Carmel; and he cast
himself down upon the earth, and put his face between his
knees' (I Kings 18, 42)

Elijah felt the need to show his humility to God, and the posture which bears his name is used frequently in hatha yoga, and is of particular relevance to yoga and prayer groups. It also plays an important part in the prayers included in this work. The attitude of the posture is a preparation for the acceptance of God's grace and a consciousness of the Spirit incarnate. (Theme of the spirituality of matter). It evokes the image of a white stone. Other postures may vary, but these are constant and irreplaceable.

The body takes the original foetal position – a test of adversity for the soul:

– The soles of the feet and palms of the hands are opened out towards the sky, from which they receive positive energy.

– This immobility and surrender renounce both sight and power, retaining only the hearing, so that interiorization is effected. The renunciation of sight calms the mind, leaving the whole being in a state of availability to the divine presence.

– The curve of the back is completely stretched, in order to free the nerve fibres between the vertebrae, and to open and spread out the vertebral discs. This eases the back.

– The nape of the neck is no longer stiff because the relevant vertebrae are stretched, which allows the energy from the heart to pass through the head, and the power of God to descend to the heart.

– The brain is oxygenaged because of the bent position.

– Breathing is gentle and regular.

– The closed body conserves the energy received through the hands and feet from the sun, the supporting surface being the earth, which also supplies energy.

– The shoulders decontract and fall.

– The body rests comfortably on the ground from which it sprang, and although it is perfectly relaxed, it is nevertheless ready to obey any call immediately.

– The kidneys, through which are filtered the sounds of God, are open, and offering themselves to the Divine Force.

– The solar plexus, centre of anxieties, is protected by the crook of the stomach.

Here is a brief example of the complementarity of body/mind/spirit, and its relation to prayer. An entire book has been written about this posture (and there are others!) for it has numerous repercussions to which particular attention should be paid.

It should be noted that in some variants, the position of the hands is modified.

– Keep the arms slightly bent.

– Or the arms may be folded to form a cross, palms away towards the sky.

– Or the hands may be clasped behind the back, one hand holding the wrist of the other.

– Or the hands are held palm to palm, against the back.

– Or the arms are stretched straight up above the head, hands joined, index fingers pointing upwards.

Each of these attitudes has a particular resonance. In general, these resonances are identical, but each individual will create and experience them in a different way. The symbolism of the body differs according to race, so the same attitude does not necessarily represent the same interior reaction. This is similar to a child being carried by his mother, either on the heart, on the hip, or on the back. In each position, the child's body receives a different rhythm, so his reactions are equally different. The vibrations which resound on the tongue develop certain regions of the self, so that the name by which parents call a child becomes a kind of mantra, which, repeated millions of time during infancy, has profound repercussions.

The Hindus have a body symbolism which differs greatly from that of Westerners, and certain Hindu mudras, or gestures of the hands, would have different repercussions when used by a Westerner. The Westerner usually prefers to keep the hands held open with the palms turned towards the sky. Nevertheless, the hatha yoga postures can lead to perceptions parallel to those of the Hindus, the pliers being an excellent example. It is said that the yogi who can hold this posture of three hours will see God. In the context of Grace, it is an evocation of the Most Holy Face. It is the belief of Hatha Yoga experts that the Hatha Yoga postures are actually imprinted in the cells of man, and that he discovers them instinctively when he achieves self-knowledge. One who at the age of six had heard neither of God nor of Hatha Yoga has had profound experiences which have resulted in *Yoga and Prayer*, which is surely a good example of the validity of this belief, and makes this work a more authentic testimony to the universal and human applications of the yoga discipline, which serves man, rather than any particular ideology or religion.

The soul can understand and communicate in ways which are impossible for the intellect. Mere words, from an intellectual source, can prove to be very limited. The Hindus have given their spirituality to Hatha Yoga, and many complain that it perverts the purity of the discipline to adapt it to the needs of Westerners. But all men are fashioned in the image of God, and by his own hand, so that all the basic laws are absolutely identical, even if the body symbolism is different. The Hindus have had the privilege of safeguarding these millenial treasures, and there is complete rapport between them and hatha yoga. The transition is simply a translation.

B. The lotus posture (J 44)

As everyone knows, the favourite posture of the Hindus is the lotus, which is usually unattainable for Westerners, who find it so necessary to compete with each other, trying to impress the neighbours and keep up with the Jones.

The half-lotus is not so difficult to master. The most important key is the possession of a stable attitude, and the ability to maintain it for a long time without strain, in order to meditate or pray. The spiritual advantages of this posture are more significant than the physical.

– As in Elijah's posture, the hands and feet are opened out towards the sky, evoking a flower, which opens its petals to the first rays of the sun, in order to receive spiritual energy.

– This posture gives stability; the equilibrium, which is stored in the lower half of the body, disposing itself so that the body is more receptive to the idea of prayer and meditation.

– The respiratory rhythm is aided, then united with the mind, which ceases to wander. The pranic energies of each side of the body circulate freely, and distribute themselves evenly.

The Hindu mystics use this posture to levitate themselves. The heels are placed one on top of the other, the upper sides of the feet being turned towards the ground in order to reduce the gential organs and to convert sexual energy into psychic energy. It is necessary to maintain the pose for a very long time before such a result may be achieved (married couples should avoid pressing the heels against the genitals).

C. The hands

During the lotus posture, or its variants, Orientals place the hands in a very special position, and traditional books teach the secrets of these mudras and their spiritual repercussions. The Hatha Yoga symbolism of the hands is just as profound and symbolic, but quite different. Many of the gestures are used in sacred biblical rites, as they receive Divine energy, and transmit it within.

The hand almost blossoms into its thumb and four fingers. The articulation of the thumb assesses force and creativity. If it is kept close to the fingers, this is an indication of introversion and reticence, whereas a thumb which is held wide apart from the fingers indicates generosity and an out-going nature. The two hands reunited (5 plus 5 equals 10) symbolize the return of unity – a meeting of both right and left sides of the body, which is a fusion of positive and negative forces. Instinctively the hands are joined in a sign of reconciliation which is outside all duality. The yogi's symbol of union with others is a bow – a typical example of contrasting corporal symbolism. Two reunited hands form a heart, or a crown, indicating the promise of a royal future, well-earned. Except for deformities from accidents or illnesses, the form of the hand is an indication of the disposition of the possessor. Sometimes the fingers are crooked, and cannot be straightened; sometimes the fingers are spread out so much that they cannot be held close together. The hand gives and receives, and its position during prayer is of the utmost significance.

The hands are held out so that the Lord may fill them with his love and they may carry it carefully to the heart, without losing a particle. The hand, symbol of creative power, is a visible continuation of the heart, which is itself a symbol of love. And is love not the greatest existing power in a world that was originally created by Him?

D. Symbolic postures

The association between prayer and the hands is the essence of the symbolic postures.

These postures produce an awareness of the bond between gestures and availability to prayer. The prayers literally seem to gush from the heart and spring spontaneously to the lips. This has been the experience of all those who have assumed the postures. They may be practised sitting, like a nun; on the knees; tailor-fashion; or flat on the stomach, as in consecration. Usually, by the end of the course, each individual has discovered the position most suited to his own temperament. The following symbol postures are very conducive to prayer:

– Arms stretched up high, giving birth to both prayer and supplication.
– If the arms are opened wide, the supplication becomes hope.
– Arms held straight down, hands open to show the palms: availability.
– Arms crossed, hands on opposite shoulders: self-communion, the attitude of Mary.
– Arms crossed, silence observed: respect for the immense suffering of Christ on the cross.
These are all postures of availability testifying to an acceptance of the

Divine Will. That Christ's death upon the cross was inevitable is symbolized by the open position, which represents a total gift.

The structure of the posture is primarily related to that of the vertical trunk of a dead tree, rooted solidly in the earth. Then a parting from the earth towards the sky is constructed; this corresponds to the constant interior of man; man centred in his original source; man's acceptance of his earthly origins. This solidity opens out horizontally like two protective wings completely stretching all the energies which fertilise humanity, giving new life to the dead tree as blood gives life to the body through feet, hands and sides. This symbolism of Christ on the Cross has an infinite number of permutations and connotations, so that extensive meditation on the subject can prove extremely fruitful and of a significance so profound that mere words are not adequate enough to describe it. For a Christian, the 'opening out' dimension of this posture expresses a welcome to the Holy Spirit, an aspect which is too often ignored by most Westerners who practise the discipline. Everyone should bear in mind the religious origins and spiritual objectives of yoga.

The cells of the body possess memories, ancestral recordings which subconsciously condition and motivate. Thus, when Occidentals deny their baptism and heritage by adopting an oriental religion, the results are frequently dissolution and narcissism. Oriental spirituality is equally oriented towards love and giving, but Westerners should adapt yoga to Christianity rather than change their religion in order to embrace yoga. Hatha Yoga is itself just such an adaptation of yoga to Christian spirituality, with the vision of availability and the image of Christ; gifts which are mutually exchanged between man and God, showing man's unity with him and reflecting the glory of his Resurrection.

From this vision and unity with Christ is born the concept of transparency – the reflection of the high waters in the low waters. Here also is pity – the infinite mercy of God, leaning forward so that his image is reflected in man! Is it possible, that in the face of such pity, anyone could not be filled with love? Man is insignificant and imperfect, but if he takes the attitudes which correspond to the animals of creation, he will acquire their characteristics; gifts given to the animals by God. Become a sheep, a dog, a grasshopper, a frog – humble creatures with more faith than man. At sunrise, listen to the sounds of nature – birdsong, animal cries, and the buzz of insect life. Listen to the grunts and clucks and yelps which greet the new day and the return of light. These are spontaneous songs of praise, being offered up by the whole of creation – except man. Man is lazing in bed, and grumbling. The humble animals are nearer their Creator than man! Mighty humanity, supported and cherished for all eternity, why do you not stretch and leap and shout with joy in the face of such patience and gentleness? No, mighty humanity prefers to degrade itself by forgetting the sacredness of the body, fouling it with grimaces and abusing it with misuse. And the abuse of the body is the abuse of self.

Different sounds produce different reactions. Some sounds are stirring and inspiring, while others are depressing. So it is with gestures – some gestures may have a very bad effect upon those who make them, whereas other gestures spiritualize the body, making it an enviable possession and inspiring in others the wish for emulation. The latter are the poetic gestures of prayer, where the discipline of yoga unites body, soul, prayer, and poetry to create music which is a cosmic vibration.

The prayers included in the text were not intellectually composed, nor were they the products of a wandering mind. They were born of the precise attitudes of body entirely inhabited by the aspirations of the soul, and of a thirst for God. Prayer sprang into being spontaneously; it was the spiritual repercussion of conscious gestures, which gushed forth like water from a mountain spring. The prayers are not intended as models to be recited verbatim, or imitated, they are simply presented as examples which should form a guideline to creative prayer. Each individual should form his own prayers, which will be invoked by the discovery of the link between body and soul.

In contrast to other works on the subject, the theme of *The Spirituality of Matter* was composed some weeks before the accompanying programme of postures was compiled. In reality, it is the story of thirty years of the author's life, reflecting a childhood spent with a family background of atheism, which created a hunger for 'something else'. The theme is an authentic account of how the body finally discovered the soul. If only the account of that experience could form a bond between writer and reader. If only the sharing of this experience were to form an invisible line of communication between them, they would be united by nature, invoking a rapport which could ultimately be transmitted to the whole of creation. Then with every sunrise, humanity would join together, and with all the other creatures offer songs of praise to God, and become collaborators in his work. Relax, and in the attitude of resurrection, make a purifying exhalation. The hands, which are united by the body, are slowly raised on an inhalation. This fortifies the whole being, as it draws in God's energy. Then, finally, the fingers slacken, the arms are stretched as far as possible, and having designed a heart in the air, they are lowered to the sides. This is the heart of Christ, the consort, full of love, shining on the whole of creation.

E. Postures of availability

While God is constantly available, man on the other hand, makes himself scarce! To live the corporal attitudes is to attain a state of availability, and to become the echo of his word – a solid entity joining earth and sky. To become available is to accept obedience, obedience implying confidence, surrender, and finally, Love.

The downfall and surrender of humanity are intimately linked with obedience. Adam knew death through disobedience. Jesus surrendered to man by dying in obedience to God's will. His attitude was entirely available, and a renunciation of himself.

Availability is an interior state which is engendered by the correct attitude of the body able to maintain it. Obedience to God is difficult, because it requires permanency, but man is constantly in a confused state, worried about his problems and divided by his interests.

In placing the body in an attitude of availability, self–knowledge is increased. These attitudes fall into a number of categories, but the following selection serve the purpose quite adequately.
– physically: solidity and balance on the ground.
– spiritually: poverty and humility of the spirit.

All Christians know that, for the believer, humility is one of the essential virtues, precious material which God is able to fashion in his way. But it is very difficult to acquire humility, much less to be born with it. Pride lies in wait for everyone, and there is the constant risk of falling into the trap. Throughout history, God has always sought out the most humble of his people. In order to accomplish his divine plan, he found that unique man Moses. God needed a man who could completely leave hold, surrender unconditionally; a man who would offer no resistance. To achieve this state, man must be 'empty' of all personal covetousness, for God will fill him with his riches, as he can trust him to keep them safe.

Man is completely conditioned by his time. Not that one epoch is really any worse than another, but contemporary life happens to be based entirely upon competition, success, and glory, objectives which hardly equate with humility. Fortunately, the Church has conserved the Psalms, which are full of adoration and humility of spirit, but alas, they are often recited without gestures. Surely the people of God should prostrate themselves – sing, dance, play the tambourine and the zither while offering up these living songs of praise? They are songs of joy and suffering, the heart's flight to God. King David did not hesitate to humble himself before Jehovah, and those who repeat his psalms should follow his example.

The postures of availability are as follows:
– The postures on the ground – lying on the back or the stomach.
– All the variants of the sitting on the ground postures.
– The upright postures of resurrection, with diverse positions of arms and hands.
– The open postures, where the heart and solar plexus are offered.

All the postures are entirely assembled on three planes – mental, physical and spiritual. They are perfectly united because both sides of the body are equally balanced. Only certain specific postures deviate from this rule.

The following sequence of simple postures express availability and humility in different ways:

- Surrender (postures of relaxation)
- Adoration (prostration)
- Welcome (open)
- Hearing (either with a straight trunk, or in a bent leaf.)
- Calling (with raised arms)
- Trust (arms crossed on the chest)

God being infinite, this is of course a limited selection, and there are many more methods and personal variants. The supply is positively inexhaustible, providing an unending source of discovery and research. When the themes have been closen:
- Being on a deep exhalation, then breathe a few more times, deeply and regularly.
- Benefit from the movements of the descent on an exhalation.
- And the movements ascending on an inhalation.
- Push the exhalation agains the hara, just above the navel. Then remount conscientiously, stage by stage.

In addition, take the following steps:
- A time of silence and surrender, in order to unite the three planes. Drop all muscular activity, and calm the mind.
- Stretch, in order to liberate the contractions of the shoulders, and put the available energy back into circulation, just as the blood circulates through the body.
- An attitude of prostration, adoration, or humility.
- An open, welcoming posture.

While maintaining a posture, breathe deeply and regularly, balancing inhalation and exhalation. In the event of hyper-activity, prolong the exhalation.

While carrying out the postures, always bear in mind the advice given in the introduction.

1. Live each posture exclusively physically, without formulating any prayer.

2. Allow the prayer to form of its own accord, invoked by the attitudes of the body.

3. Introduce living prayer during the postures, without praying verbally.

The proposed series of sequenced movements will have repercussions from the resulting union of the three planes – physical, mental and spiritual; the repercussions operate rather like the domino principle, where one will ricochet off the other. But the real value of this unity is the repercussion between God and man. Man should resemble a receptive wall, of which bounces an echo, and whose transparent surface reflects the sky. If he does not, then the unification of the planes has limitations.

Research has indicated that the different spatial attitudes of the human body pass beyond these attitudes, so that the initial rapport between the three planes creates a personal rapport. Man, at peace with himself, finds that his new sense of wholeness is transmuted into a wholeness with God.

Spatially, man's position is between earth and sky. He obtains negative energy from the earth and positive energy from the sun. The unison of these two forces provides him with the energy he needs.

In the postures of availability, the attitudes of the body will differ, according to their order in the sequences. There are multiple structures for these attitudes, and each individual will be able to discover new aspects and patterns. One attitude will evolve from another, any modification depending upon the basic position – upright; lying down; sitting. Eventually, the development may lead to a completely different attitude, or to another starting-point which may take a different direction. The cycle can either be finished, or left open for more complex and intense composition. There are, however, three invariables:
– the earth; the sky; the upright position, without any rigidity of the spinal column.
Variable elements are:
– The position of the arms, through a rapport with fixed points.
– The position of the hands, opened out towards the sky, towards the earth, or joined together.
– The position of the head.
– The arrangement of the body.

The disposition of the variable elements is of course to a certain extent limited, as man cannot escape from his origins. But however resourceful man becomes, however far he pushes himself, tries to break records, or defy natural laws, his true vocation is the service of God on earth. Man is the child of God, and he can only fulfil this role through the fusion of mind, body, and spirit, for only this will make him available to his Father.

POSTURES OF AVAILABILITY

Sitting–on–the–ground

(All variants)

Either spend some time on the development of a single posture, or develop several to make up a new cycle.

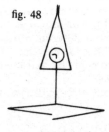

fig. 48

1. (First, exhale thoroughly, joining the hands in prayer)

purification
mental calm

2. Liberation from all egotism

stretching
liberation
fortifying
inhalation

fig. 49

3. In order to reflect his image

opening
welcoming
reconstruction of the back

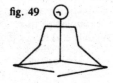

fig. 50

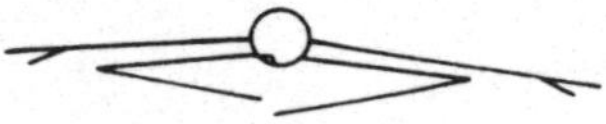

4. Welcoming his will

opening
surrender
obedience
hearing

fig. 51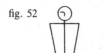

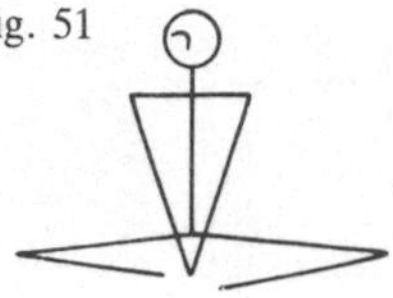

1. Advance towards him

stretching
and bowing
and inhaling

fig. 52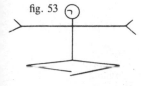

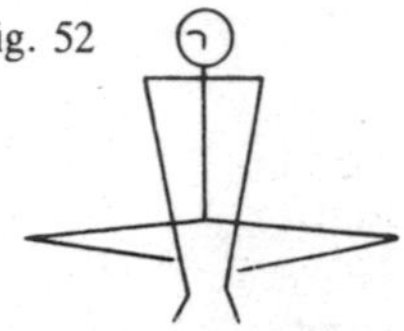

2. In order to be filled with his love

reconstruct the back, rise, open out.
Bracing
inhalation

fig. 53

3. Open out to others

bow in a gesture of welcome, the arms wide open.
surrender
obedience
humility
purifying exhalation

fig. 54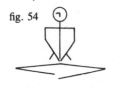

4. Welcome the graces with which he fills man

second stretching on an exhalation.
relaxation
surrender

·5. Bringing those graces to the heart

reconstruction of the back.
listening
posture

fig. 55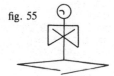

6. In order to make them bear fruit

attention
trust

POSTURES STARTING ON THE STOMACH

I. Simple sequence: from the lying position to the sitting position.

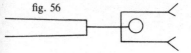

fig. 56

Take me to my rest,
Take me to myself.

relaxation
surrender
stretching
unification

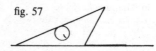

fig. 57

Lead me into your light so
that all will be peaceful and
clear.

stretching
humility
supplication
preparation of the back

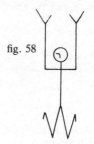

fig. 58

No longer accept my departure from your ways,
Let my attention not turn
from you

opening
welcoming
conscious
presence
listening
reconstruction of the verte
bral support

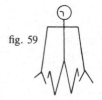

fig. 59

Let me live near you

attention
trust
perfect attitude
not stiff
not relaxed

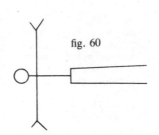

fig. 60

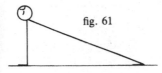

fig. 61

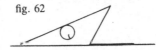

fig. 62

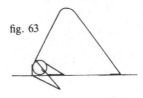

fig. 63

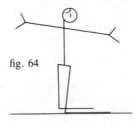

fig. 64

II

1. I belong to You
   I surrender myself to you

relaxation
surrender
decontraction
unification

2. Towards you I aspire, towards you I direct my thoughts

stretching
supplication
bracing inhalation twice
mount on inhalation
descend on exhalation

3. In order to serve you

preparation of the back
prostration
purifying exhalation

4. In all humility

reverse posture
humility
oxygenation of the brain
balanced inhalation and exhalation

5. I open myself out to you in order to reflect your image

opening
welcoming
recharge through the plexus
bracing posture

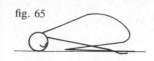

fig. 65

6. Keeping your image in my heart

relaxing the back
open limbs turned towards the sky
mind soothed by means of closed eyes
listening to the word

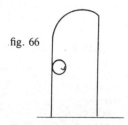

fig. 66

7. Hearing you call; responding to your voice.

second preparation of the back
stretching
surrender

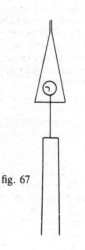

8. When your Spirit raises me upright.

complete vertical reconstruction
hands open, therefore receptive

fig. 67

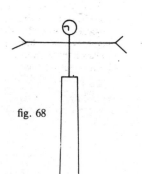

9. A testament to your glory.

availability
equilibrium
solidity of the hara
balanced inhalation and exhalation

fig. 68

10. Towards the accomplishment of your work.

complete opening in the perfect attitude, balanced and solid

POSTURES COMMENCING IN AN UPRIGHT POSITION: NEHEMIAH

(Nehemiah, chapter 8)

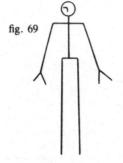

fig. 69

1. And all the people gathered themselves together as one man . . . (8, 1)

(i) Return to unity

2. And Ezra opened the book in the sight of all the people, (for he was above all the people) and when he opened it, all the people stood up (8, 5)

(ii) Man becomes a sounding board, echoing the word of God. He is receptive and attentive to the sound, and stable and solid in his relation to the ground. He gathers together all the energies which connect earth and sky.

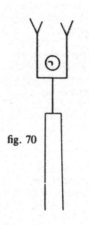

fig. 70

3. And Ezra blessed the Lord, the Great God. And all the people answered Amen, Amen, with lifting up their hands: (8, 6).

(iii) Maximum stretching of the spinal column. The circulation of the energy is activated. Well-anchored to the ground, man manifests his desire to discover anew his divine vocation. His hands, precious gift of the Creator, wishing to associate his child with his works, raise him up towards the Father, and he receives positive energy. Approbation; giving; hope.

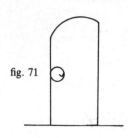

fig. 71

4. . . . and they bowed
their heads . . . (8, 6)

After stretching, the
back is massaged and
relaxed. Submission;
acceptance; humility;
recall of earthly origins;
surrender; trust; respect.

fig. 72

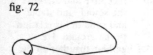

5. . . . and worshipped the
Lord with their faces to
the ground (8, 6).

(v) Man returns to his
original form, which is
that of a seed. Once
again, he possesses the
spirit of a child. After
having received the
word, man allows himself
to ripen by means of the
negative energy to which
he surrenders himself.
Meanwhile, he is
completely available to
God.

Complete
submission; an
acceptance of the
imperfections of the
world.

IV PRAYER AND THE BODY

THE SPIRITUALITY OF MATTER, OR THE CONCEPT OF BEING

1. PRAYERS

Prayer: I will become a new–born *lamb*, as in the days of my youth when I came out of Egypt. You will carry me on your shoulders, and I will be strengthened by the rhythm of your steps. You will join me to yourself for all eternity, because your love transcends all others.
Posture: Position of relaxation; a child sleeping on its side (A2).

Prayer: When I am fully grown, you will set me down on all fours, and I shall have the strength of a *lion* of Judah, but the cattle will still come to graze at my side.
Posture: Position of a lion, without extending the tongue; legs crossed.

Prayer: I shall be a *servant* of the Most-High, and my ears will await your commands. I feel you around me, Lord, and I surrender myself to the perfume of your presence. I place my trust in the calm of repose, and I shall be ready for your call.
Pity me! Pity me! Give me the gift of your mercy!
Posture: Muslim prayer position; completely stretched out like a cat or a dog (G29).

Prayer: If you wish, I shall become a humble *cricket*, nourishing myself with the rays of the burning sun, which is a symbol of your power. I shall eternally sing the hymn of life; both by night and by day the celestial arch will ring with the sound of my voice, so that all creation will know of my love for you.
Posture: Inhale and exhale on all fours, one bent leg raised at the back, knee against the thigh.

Prayer: I will be the courageous *hero*, for deep in me is rooted justice, and your name is inscribed upon my chest. I shall not flee from my enemies, and they will read your name and know that you are my beloved,

that your arms are powerful, and you are unique. Lord, they will learn that you are perfection.
Posture: Hero position (F18).

Prayer: Your gifts dazzle me, Lord, and I reflect them, becoming a glittering *diamond* with a million facets which reflect your glory. I will burn with all the fires of creation, Lord, for I am made in your image.
Posture: Diamond position (F17).

Prayer: I will be as a white *pebble*, a rolling stone which brings a new name to those who have not heard it, and they will know it as the name of victory. This will be done, Lord, through your all-powerful mercy.
Pity me! Pity me! Give me the gift of your mercy!
Posture: Bent leaf (G30).

Prayer: And the white pebble shall become a *mountain*, for I shall be raised up by his love, and my love shall dwell there. O you mountains and hills, bless the Lord! The creatures who climb you come to hear his word; bless them!
Posture: Attitude of watching the sunrise.

Prayer: Remembering my errors, at each season, like a *serpent* I shall strip myself of my old garments. Thus will I redeem myself, for my faults will be erased. Pity me! Pity me! Give me the gift of your mercy!
Posture: Cobra, flat on the stomach, hands behind the back.

Prayer: Now I shall be a humble *grasshopper* and devastate the field of my sins. All shall be cut down, not one shall escape me. My sins shall be destroyed, for the fire of your love will devour them, leaving a desolate desert upon which the Garden of Eden will reflower.
Posture: F20 or 21.

Prayer: I will become *Noah's ark*, and the animals will be my friends. I will live in communion with them, and from the sky above us will shine your radiance. The earth and all its creatures will be bathed in the Light of your love, and a dove will bring me an olive branch!
Pity me! Pity me!
Posture: Noah's ark: F22. The dove: F24.

Prayer: My joy will be so great that I shall be as light as a *gazelle*. My ankles are slender, but so strong that I shall fill the forests with my grace. I will bound over mountains! I will leap over hills, following my course without pause or rest!
Posture: I36.

Prayer: If it is your wish, I will make myself as small as a friendly *frog*. Joyful and ignorant, I will reclaim the waters of the sky, and be purified.
Posture: I33.

Prayer: I will beg for your love, and you will transform me into a *star*. Now, resplendent as morning, I will possess the splendour you had wished to be mine! The mantle of your royalty will descend upon me, and I will become your queen, as you are my king. Your face will be my light! All creation prostrates itself before you!

Pity me! Pity me! Give me the gift of your mercy!

Posture: G27.

Prayer: My wings glittering and glowing with your splendour, I shall flit from flower to flower in the form of a *dragonfly*, and I will gather there the nectar of their hearts and offer it to you.

Posture: On the back, hands under the nape of the neck. Inhale and exhale while moving the arms like wings.

Prayer: The sweetness of my offering meets your power as it enters into me, and I shall be as a *crocodile*. My breath will shine with the light from my scales, which form a wall of shields, so that no flesh is able to reach me. I will lie under the lotus, and even if the river rages, I shall not be disturbed.

Posture: Gentle twisting of the torso while lying on the back. Arms held straight above the head.

Prayer: Like the *tortoise*, I shall know when to retreat into myself. Ignoring the illusions of false gods, I shall be resurrected by your word, making my way without useless haste.

Pity me! Pity me! Bestow on me the gift of your mercy!

Posture: G28.

Prayer: And this life, which lies buried deep in my innermost being, will gush out towards the heights. I will lift myself up like an *eagle*, and live in the summits of the cliffs. Lifting the little ones aloft, I will look around and discover the mysteries of your works and the extent of your love.

Posture: I35.

Prayer: I will contemplate in all its glory the *tree* upon which your only Son has given himself. He has transformed the dead trunk of the tree into eternal life, bequeathing me his divine heritage, by which I am redeemed.

Posture: I37.

Prayer: At last I shall be able to sit in your shadow, just as a wife waits for her husband. I will be like a *lily*, and your name will be on my forehead. You will again make me as pure as I was on the day when you breathed your breath into my nostrils and gave me life. You will say to me: 'Come, because you are thirsty for the water of life!' And there will no longer be any night, for you will shine on me for all eternity. The verdant tree will be my dwelling, and clapping my hands, I will proclaim your name and your glory from the topmost branches, and all will find a niche in your kingdom.

Pity me! Pity me! You are the God of mercy!
Posture: Sitting-on-the-ground posture.

2. MEDITATION

This is the extraordinary story of the relationship between the body and the soul, and the eventual spiritualization of the soul. It is the story of the conquest of the body by the aspirations of the soul. It is a spark, sent down by the Almighty, so that others may be warmed by his fire and illuminated by his love.

In the beginning, man was an unformed mass, lying on the ground. Then the mass left the ground. It was of the earth, it entered time and space, it was washed by the sea, sheltered by the sky and warmed by fire – it became part of the world. It contained life; it lived.

1. *Lotus, or waist bent and head bowed in prayer, arms behind the back.*

This living organism awoke, explored the world, touched it, became familiar with it, and resolved to conquer it. But to conquer the world is to conquer the body, for is the body not part of the world? So a choice had to be made. Conquer the world, and cripple the body? Or use the body as a springboard to attain – what? Somewhere in the darkness a faint spark glittered feebly. What was it? Intangible, almost indiscernible, yet it existed, conveying a profound sense of being the source of all things. Man was tempted to rise up and go forth, to seek for what lay beyond; to discover the source!

2 *Arms open; hands on the ground forming a half-circle, then rejoining in front of the head.*

3 *Supported on the back in a foetus.*

But the body did not wish to leave the earth, and the body was strong. The life within wished to make an alliance with the body it inhabited; It wished to be faithful to the body, and to be in accord with the body, so at first it simply served the body. It explored and inquired and satisfied the body's curiosity. Then, having found what was at the bottom of everything, the body wondered what was to be found at the top.

4 *Head descends, to be held in the hands.*

5 *The feet are raised.*

6 *Then slowly lowered.*

A great force came from on high, (*the candle*) it combined with the rhythm of life to develop all the life on the earth, so that it bloomed and grew (*dynamic phase of the candle*).

The feeble spark of the soul felt the force from on high, and blossomed. Thus, it was able to support the body. It followed the soothing and strengthening rhythm of the sun, which guides all creation and is a witness to his love which created all things. So the soul took the body to dwell with him, to receive the total gift – to discover his love, which can have no equal.

7 *Chariot (E13).*

8 *Balanced candle.*

But the body wished to return to the earth from which it had parted, to return to its origins, to find a refuge, and to rest before setting out again on its pilgrimage into space.

9 *Stick: the body is flat on the ground.*

The soul took the body north, south, east and west, like waves going out from the garden of Eden.

10 *Twisting while lying on the ground.*

This mysterious labour of the human soul is the slow progression of the spiritualization of the body.

11 *Half-pliers (J42)*

So that finally the body may become the soul, and fly away with it.

12 *Boat (I34). Torso and legs rise, body supported only by the buttocks.*

The force which merges body with soul is the same force which initially breathed life into the body, animating it, and binding it to all creation, where it pulses and breathes without ceasing.

12 *Ditto, then with legs bent, the body slides forward.*

This is the breath of God, which aspires to higher things, and so sweeps the body into a state of prayer.

13 *Cobra on one knee, arms in air, hands joined in prayer.*

The effort, the struggle, transmigration – all must be accepted.

14 *Reverse bow (F23).*

An awareness of the Spirit Incarnate will bring the soul back to the body.

15 *Bent leaf (F30).*

The soul is free to choose a perpetual return to the earth from whence it came.

16 *Posture on the head, or reversed, following the dolphin. Return to bent leaf, fists under forehead.*

The body and the soul are ultimately unified by the glory of the Creator of all that was and ever will be.

17 *Upright, hands joined, one leg slightly back.*

Man makes a final mystical union with his infinite surroundings.

18 *Tree, hands arched above the head.*

V THE BASIS OF A HEALTHY DIET

During the preliminary stages, before beginning the asanas, traditional yoga attends to the purity of the body at different levels, one of these being a diet which fits due preparation for spiritual exercises.

Diet has a very important influence upon an individual's behaviour, and has profound repercussions on his or her spiritual life. Hatha yoga is particularly concerned with diet, for the energies of the body are internally nourished by the ingestion of food and by respiration, and the progress of yoga discipline is activated by this nourishment. Food has a negative element, which is transformed into human cells. The quality of the blood is directly attributable to the quality of the food ingested, so that a corresponding quality of activity will be produced.

Respiration carries a positive element, bringing vital oxygen to the blood cells, and if the breathing is good the cells will be conditioned and invigorated. The different elements of man are complementary. An excessive diet and inadequate respiration will result in an imbalance and an unhealthy structure, the organism being both deprived and throttled.

Illness is not a punishment, but nature's alarm signal. Illness does not conform to the law of harmony, and that it should represent some form of punishment from God is to the Christian a particularly alien concept. God is all love, and illness is more of a precious sign, placed in the organism so that any erratic behaviour may be corrected.

Dietetic errors are so numerous that a number of systems have been devised and a number of organizations established for the sole purpose of dealing with the problem. No doubt they are all sincere in their intentions, but they all disagree! This is rather discouraging to the layman, who finally abandons his quest for a healthy diet and returns to his usual bad habits. Actually, most schools of thought base their systems upon established fact, so that they are bound to be correct in some respects.

But people do not respond in the same way to the same diet, and this is where the yogi has an advantage over the non-yogi. It is evident that dietary problems are best resolved by the intelligence of the body rather than by the intellect itself, so the subject must be de-intellectualized. The natural wisdom of the body can be brought into play by means of yoga discipline. This wisdom is stored in the memory cells, and is a precious natural instinct. Yoga is a stripping of all superfluous matter, giving an appreciation of true values. A diet should be selected according to the judgment of the individual, based on this same 'stripping' principle. The objective is a simple, unadulterated diet. Mother Nature placed deep breathing and diet hand-in-hand, in order to produce harmony and balance.

Live according to nature's directions, and begin by observing nature. Everyone knows what an uncanny ability the human mother seems to acquire when she has the responsibility of feeding her young. Similarly, the Creator has provided for man, each season bringing its own crop of nourishment. So diet is a question of love between God and man, but man has corrupted this. Christians will surely recognize the importance accorded to food throughout the Scriptures. Some of the greatest events in the New Testament take place against the background of some feast or repast, such as the wedding at Cana; the return of the Prodigal Son; many feast days; and the Last Supper, the Holy Communion. After the Resurrection, Jesus himself prepared a meal for the disciples by the side of the lake.

Diet is an important aspect of the life of each individual, whether believer or non-believer. Any departure from the natural order should be considered wrong, and everyone should sincerely try to restore balance and harmony to the diet. A yogi knows that he should shun all mechanical behaviour. He knows that a course of postures and a complete system of respiration will give him the ability to observe, concentrate, and use his judgment. No quick canteen meals for him! He may eat less food, but it is better food, and he takes full advantage of the energy transmitted to the body by each mouthful; the pranic energy which is drawn in by respiration is also found in food. Nobody is suggesting 'the drinking of food and chewing of liquids', but mastication should be improved. Some authorities suggest a count of 50–100 for each mouthful, but it is easier simply to savour the food thoroughly, keeping it soaked for as long as possible in those secretions which nature has provided for the purpose of preparing the stomach, which in its turn produces secretions sent by the intestines. Mass-produced adulterated food should always be avoided.

Non-believers are renewed by the great energetic laws of *prana*, while believers are renewed by grace and prayer. It is in the mouth that the wonderful transformation of good takes place – it becomes human cells, so obviously the manner in which the food is eaten has great significance. Man lives upon what he digests, not what he ingests. Some suggest that 'we are what we eat', but surely man is better than what he eats?

HOW TO CHOOSE A DIET

The yogi certainly knows the answer to the question 'How do I choose what I eat?' because yoga discipline has taught him the wisdom of nature. Whenever possible he eats the produce of his own country, choosing whenever possible the fruits and vegetables which are in season. He eats simply, but wisely. Cereals may be eaten all the year round, as they can be preserved without additives, but all out-of-season produce which has been chemically treated should be avoided. This is a plus rather than a minus; not a deprivation, but a beneficial alternative. Take pity on the headaches, the liver troubles, the coughs and the colds! Change to a healthy diet – and that does not necessarily mean a diet exclusive of all delicious food or an end to enjoyable meals. Food is of itself a pleasure, and justly so, as it supports life. A Christian knows that all the meals in the New Testament were joyful occasions. Unfortunately, most modern foods are adulterated by chemical additives, with the result that perfectly good natural produce is rendered tasteless and harmful. A yogi is able to savour and enjoy a mouthful of good bread and a swallow of pure water. It is always a good idea to observe the demeanour of those who advocate any special diet. Of course, even an appearance of sparkling health does not prove the efficacy of any diet, but at least it is a good indication.

Nature is no fanatic, and she is good-natured enough not to make man answerable for occasional lapses in the area of diet. She has foresight, and builds up a high level of tolerance to harmful substances, otherwise man would not last very long.

Age, occupation, background, heredity and aspirations are all factors which play a part in assessing the nourishment most suitable and necessary for the individual. Nobody should attempt to lay down the law or imagine that he has said the last word on the subject of diet. Everyone should discover his own ideal diet by means of trial and error, for it must depend upon life-style and physique. It is impossible to solve the diet problems of others, but it is possible to pass on the results of personal experience, research, and experiment, in the hope that they will prove helpful. The suggestions made here should be adapted, using judgment and instinct.

The following diet has proved to be very healthy:

Midday
seasonable fruits and vegetables.
an egg, or fish, or vegetable pâté, or some vegetable dish.
cereals
cheese

Evening
steamed or braised vegetables.
milk pudding (such as semolina or tapioca)
stewed fruit
or

soup (thickened with cereals or rice)
cheese
sea-weed dessert

In winter, eat more cereals, but in spring, reduce the amount of cereal and replace it with seasonable vegetables. In summer, reduce both cereals and vegetables, replacing them with seasonable fruits. This is not a hard-and-fast rule, simply a guide-line.

Preferably, fruits and vegetables should be eaten at the beginning of or during a meal, so that they will be digested quickly, and not ferment in the stomach. For the same reason, it is advisable to fast in the morning. Meat may be eaten, but not too much. A little poultry is preferable. But the results of a six-year vegetarian diet have proved so excellent that those who feel able to undertake it would be advised to do so. The articulations become more supple, and there is a distinct improvement in the hatha yoga postures, particularly the lotus, which proves that the body becomes detoxified. Annoying ailments of long standing, such as pains in the shoulders and elbows, completely vanish. These findings are based upon personal experience – even otitis, which had struck several times previous to the vegetarian diet, completely disappeared. But the most notable benefit is a spiritual and mental peace, hitherto unimaginable, especially in this day and age. This is certainly the best reason to continue to be a vegetarian.

Naturally enough, meditation and prayer burgeon in this new mental and spiritual peace, and although it would be foolish to claim that it is necessary to be a vegetarian in order to pray or meditate, it certainly has a profound effect upon the inner being and illuminates the truth.

Good bread is the first priority in a healthy diet. In natural organic bread, the yeast content is high, and this is a very important factor. Never buy bread which is non-organic, even if it looks brown. It should be labelled organic, otherwise it may simply be ordinary white processed bread with which bran has been mixed before baking. This means that the finished product will contain toxic matter, and the bread will lack the essential grains. If cereals are not included in the diet, organic bread is of particular importance. Adequate literature dealing with the subject of bread and nutrition may be found elsewhere in plenty; suffice it to say here that good natural organic bread is infinitely better than mass-produced products with chemical additives.

'The right to be ill' is itself a symptom of the times – 'The right to be healthy' would be a much more logical claim. Busy, hard-working people should concentrate upon health, not upon illness. Children should be concerned with building a sound constitution. Bread is a basic food, so it can play a large part in changing attitudes to illness, as well as contributing to health. In answer to the obvious comment that organic bread is expensive, it may be pointed out that it need rarely be wasted. Processed bread becomes stale and inedible very quickly, whereas organic bread lasts longer, and may be used for puddings, soups, delicious vegetable pâtés, or simply croûtons, which give solidity to soups and vegetable purées. Bread being the first basic food in a natural healthy diet, cereals may be described as the first basic alternative.

It would be impossible to count all the benefits to be gained from the consumption of rice. But it is interesting to note that its ratio of

$$\frac{\text{potassium} \quad K}{\text{sodium} \quad Na}$$

is equal to 5, a figure near to that of the human blood. If the ratio contained much more potassium than sodium it would cause nerve trouble, passivity and dispersion, making it comparable to the potato. Rice renews and purifies the blood, thereby curing a number of maladies.

Millet, an African cereal, and buckwheat, a cereal grown in cold countries, both provide plenty of energy, as do maize, barley, and oats. Cereals are obtainable in the following forms: grains, flakes, flour, and a finely ground flour which is more adaptable and digestible for children and invalids. Corn is found in the form of couscous, semolina, biscuits and bread.

Attention must be drawn to the complementarity between vegetables and man. This complementarity is evident at the oxygen/carbon level; the tree is the best partner to humanity. But less appreciated is the fact that vegetables contain all that man needs to sustain life.

For some people, meat is a necessity, and, to prevent aggressiveness (unless it is producing any obviously bad effects), it may be eaten in moderation. After all, Hitler was a vegetarian! The more the yoga discipline is practised, the easier will it be to reduce the consumption of meat. Total abstinence is not necessary, simply the awareness and avoidance of excess. An excess of meat, like an excess of anything else, is always prejudicial, because quantity modifies quality. In supposing meat to be indispensable to the maintenance of man's life, the subject becomes dramatic. Countless animals are bred in conditions akin to those in concentration camps, fed on hormones, and expected to supply rich healthy meat! How can frightened and unhappy creatures who are full of toxins possibly provide man with healthy nourishing food? From the point of view of world hunger, it should be noted that to raise an animal for slaughter takes seven times more ground than to grow the equivalent amount of nourishment in cereals. So world hunger is linked to the corruption of world diet, and not in the least attributable to nature's lack of foresight; nature has made adequate provision for mankind. Just as peace in the world begins in the heart of the individual, the problem of world hunger is caused by the diet of each individual, a diet composed of excess and waste – particularly of meat. Those who decide to reduce their meat consumption should also reduce their sugar consumption, above all of white sugar. Sugar reduces a vitamin found in meat; too much eaten with a small amount of meat will considerably reduce your own vitamin reserves. This is why so many vegetarians, trying to make up their losses on sweetstuffs, actually lose nourishment and fall ill. Always take brown sugar and natural honey, but in moderate quantities. It is not difficult to acquire the habit of drinking tea, coffee, or herb teas without sugar. Most needs are dictated by the mind, so when it is clear that processed, chemically treated foods are having a bad effect upon the body, the intelligence of mind and of body should combine to reject all adulterated foodstuffs.

In the area of liquid nutrition, 'juice-abuse' should be avoided. It is not necessary to absorb any juice in addition to the required amount of fruit and vegetable matter; it is simply an alternative. The wisdom of nature foresaw the complementarity of the whole of creation, so all the necessities of life are natural and obtainable. Herbs are literally one of the marvels of nature, and a number of works have been written on this subject alone. The humble herb is evidence of the manifestation of the wisdom of nature. In discovering the remarkable properties of herbs, discover too the gift of love freely offered by God.

Herbs may be dried, ground, and used as spices. They purify the system, and above all, for the meat-eater, they combat decay. Formerly, spices were used in embalming processes, and they are drunk in the form of tisanes, but without sugar, as the sugar reduces the effects of the herbs. Herb teas should be drunk between or after meals. As far as tea coffee are concerned – quality counts, so drink only the best. Coffee should be light chestnut brown in colour; bad quality coffee is dark because it has been roasted to the maximum to increase the aroma, which also happens to increase the caffeine content. A good coffee does not need to be decaffeinated, because it actually contains very little caffeine, and this small amount is less dangerous than the products used for decaffeination. Macrobiotic tea is of excellent quality, as it has been allowed to dry on the branch for three years so that it loses its volatile elements. It is not strong, but boiling it twice will increase the strength. For those who fast, it is a very good appetite suppressant.

The best solution to the problem of how to avoid commercially-grown fruits and vegetables, which are sprayed with insecticides, is quite clearly the cultivation of a kitchen garden! But this being an impossibility for most people, the next best thing is to find those shops where home-grown produce is sold. The snag here is that the consumer is open to exploitation, as shopkeepers frequently triple the price of a commodity simply in order to convince the customer of its superior quality. Of course, a reputable dealer who values his customers will not do this, and a careful study of all the available shops will usually show where the best market gardeners send their produce. So many farmers try to force too much out of the land by using unnatural methods, and it is this which reduces the quality of their produce. But some conscientious farmers refuse to exhaust the land in this way, and should there be any difficulty in tracking down their retail outlets, nutritional journals are usually happy to supply information about the locations of the farmers themselves. The future of the earth, which looks after mankind, is the concern of mankind, and most sincere farmers who love the earth, and nourish and respect it, would welcome consultations with consumers.

Choice of a suitable greengrocer should not be made solely on the grounds of the beauty of his display! Carefully polished and arranged produce may present an attractive appearance and catch the eye, but it may well prove to be of inferior quality. Always wash fruit very carefully before eating it, making sure that the water is not dirty or contaminated. Everyone must resign himself to the fact that at one time or another he will be consuming a certain amount of polluted matter – the world itself is polluted, so this is unavoidable. But your organism must be accustomed to dealing with this pollution, otherwise you could never eat away from home and, in the event of an accident, even a spell in hospital would prove dangerous in itself, as the body would have an adverse reaction to all commercial products.

Equal care should be taken to wash dried fruit thoroughly, and it should be allowed to dry in the air. Although health food stores have a very good selection of dried fruits they are usually rather expensive, but they do replace sweets and snacks – 'junk food' adulterated by chemical products. Dried fruit is very good for growing children. In a simple diet where the meat consumption has been considerably reduced, 'little treats' may be introduced without any alarming consequences to the budget! They may seem expensive, but in the long run they will produce an improvement in health, and their nutritional value will far exceed that of apparently cheaper adulterated foods. And the gas bill will be lower!

In a balanced diet, oil and fat are two factors which should not be disregarded. Olive oil (from Europe) and ground nut oil (from Africa) are both excellent, but should be 100% pure, and from a first pressing. Vegetable oils of similar quality do exist, but in some shops olive oil may be purchased at comparable prices. Vegetable oil is lighter, and as so little is needed, more economical. Always 'shop around' and compare prices before making any purchases. So often, the divergence in prices of identical products can be quite astronomical.

Table salt being a dead product, sea salt should always be used instead. Cooking utensils should always be cast-iron, never use aluminium. Oven ware should be earthenware or heat-resistant glass, such as Pyrex.

Creation is all one, and no part of it may be dissociated from the others without a resulting imbalance. Nature is complementary, and man being a part of nature, he also is complementary. His three levels of spirit, mind, and physique are all linked, and they react to diet. The digestive system is linked to the nervous system, which is linked to the psyche of the individual. A malfunctioning digestive system will obviously have unfortunate repercussions.

The absorption of irritating foodstuffs, inadequate mastication, and overeating all use too much energy for digestive purposes. All this is unlikely to lead to inner consciousness and self-knowledge. But a balanced diet can cure the bad effects of modern life, and help create a better self. The tree of life should be erected vertically in man, relating him both to earth and sky. When he is available to open out towards others with a gesture of giving and love, then the world will be saved from its misery.

RECIPES

Here are a number of recipes which will provide a guideline for a simple and wholesome diet.

Cereals will prove to be very versatile and adaptable for creative cookery. Remember that the kitchen is no longer the place where the stomachs of the family are to be refilled, but rather the place where their health is to be restored and maintained by good, simple, balanced meals. None of the enjoyment should be lost – on the contrary, it should increase. Elaborate menus are not necessary; complete satisfaction and pleasure will be provided naturally – by nature.

Cereals

Rice should be cooked in a small iron saucepan with a lid.
– 1 cup rice
– 2½ cups water
Wash and sort the rice while the water comes to the boil. Throw in the rice. Allow to simmer until all the water is absorbed. Spices or herbs and salt to taste should be added shortly before the rice is cooked. Place in a covered dish in the oven. Serve with butter sauces, parsley, saffron, grated cheese, beaten egg, or mixed vegetables. With shrimp and artichoke hearts, it makes an excellent paella. Any left-over rice may be used to thicken vegetable soup. Rice, like all other cereals, is very adaptable, and may be used in a number of different dishes. It can be carried on a picnic in a thermos flask, and is very useful as it can be prepared in advance for an evening meal, when the cook may be exhausted after a hard day's work.

Millet and buckwheat

1 cup cereal
3 cups salted water
Boil the salted water in a casserole on a high flame, spoon in the millet or buckwheat, stirring occasionally until all the water has evaporated. Buckwheat should be eaten in winter.

Husked millet is recommended for sedentary people and intellectuals because it provides the system with assimilable phosphorus. It is good for students. Buckwheat is recommended for those who suffer from dilatation of the cells, or cellulitis, as the positive polarity makes a food which strengthens the cells.

Barley: grain, or ground

Soak some hours before cooking, overnight if possible.
4 parts water to 1 of cereal.
Barley has always been famous for its excellent properties as a food, and for its therapeutic value. Unfortunately, modern housekeepers are unaware of the extent of its virtues. It is less rich in nitrates than corn, and more easily tolerated by delicate systems. Its viscous consistency is helpful in all cases of inflammation of the digestive and excretory system. It is refreshing, laxative, and diuretic. It may be used as a tisane – barleywater – or made into gruel or added to soup. Before adding to soup, always pour off the water in which the barley has been soaking. Instructions for rice are also applicable to barley.

Maize is best known in the form of pop-corn. It makes a light but substantial breakfast. It may be eaten on the cob. When raw, it activates the function of the liver. It may be boiled or grilled.

Semolinas

Couscous
Cook as millet or buckwheat, but with 1½ cups of water. Boil five minutes, then when cooked, stir in little oil, to prevent sticking.
Semolina of rice; maize; barley.
If roasted, and of good quality, cook as couscous. If not, cook in two or three parts of water.

Flakes

Use in soups. For the preparation of sweet milk puddings, flakes are preferable to grains (rice or barley). Oat flakes make delicious muesli. Allow them to stand in cold milk, then mix in raisins and any seasonable fruit, except orange or lemon.

Flours

Flour is used for pancakes, patés, soups, croquettes, bread, chapatis, biscuits, pastry and so on. For children and invalids, pre-digested flours are more easily assimilable, and are used in the preparation of gruel.

Creamed cereals may be added to this gruel and eaten for breakfast, lunch or dinner, with or without vegetables.

Flour is used in thickening soups and sauces. Béchamel, a white cream sauce, is served with vegetables which have been browned in the oven with cheese and breadcrumbs. It is quite simple to invent delicious and original recipes for sauces.

– purée of carrots, or pumpkin (red sauce)
– purée of radish tops (green sauce)
– grated cheese
– soya sauce (available in bottles in all macrobiotic stores)
– chopped parsley
– sliced onion
– mushrooms, sea-weed

Chapatis may be made from flour which has not been over-refined. Make a dough with water, flour, and salt. Roll out to the thickness of a pie crust and cut into sections three or four inches square. Cook slowly, in oil if desired.

For buckwheat croquettes mix buckwheat flour, water and salt to a thick consistency: i.e., of paint. Wheat flour may be mixed with the buckwheat. Add some olive oil to the mixture, then fry in hot oil. Each dollop of the mixture should form a circular patty which is cooked on both sides on a low flame. You can mix the dough with chopped onion, chopped olives, mushrooms, vegetables, or sage cooked for ten minutes in boiling water.

Conservation of stored cereals

Untreated cereals are easily contaminated by weevils. Do not store cereals in hermetically sealed containers as weevils like neither air nor light and would be delighted to find themselves shut away in a closed receptacle. They do not like the smell of garlic, onion, or pepper, so add these to any stock of cereal. However, if any maggots should appear, bring the cereals out into the air then cook them, either in the oven or on top of the stove. The weevils will then come to the surface, and are easily removed.

Polenta

Fry some vegetables, then cover them with flour or cream of maize (polenta). After adding water to obtain a creamy consistency, cook in a casserole in a slow oven.

Corn: stoneground or pre-cooked

Boil 2½ cups salted water, and cook for 20 minutes in a covered pan on a low flame. All the water should be absorbed. Make some Béchamel sauce, mix with the corn, and freeze. When firm, cut into pieces, roll in sesame seeds or breadcrumbs and fry. Serve with a *purée* of vegetables or a sauce to taste.

Flaked cereal escalopes – corn, barley, rye, etc.

Throw the flakes into boiling salted water or soup and cook until thick. The preparation will be easier to freeze if the flakes are grilled before throwing them into the liquid. Add a little flour if the consistency is not firm enough.

Alternative additions: chopped onions and mushrooms, chopped olives, or vegetables.

Cut the preparation into slice and fry like escalopes. Serve with haricot or lentil puree.

Semolina of maize

Cream of maize, or maize flour.

Add to cooking vegetables, or minced onion. Add spices such as nutmeg or coriander. After cooking, add beaten egg or grated cheese. Turn out on to a plate, and place in the oven to heat.

Grilled buckwheat

Add flour, cooked chopped onion, cooking wine and water. Mix, then cut and cook as escalopes.

Or: Mix 8 oz buckwheat flour with ¼ pint of water, 4 oz flour and 5 spoons of yeast (optional) to obtain the consistency of thick paint. Knead in shallots, cooked onion, chopped parsley and chopped black olives. Fry in oil.

Corn escalopes

Soak the corn in water for some hours. Cook over a low flame or in the oven, adding carrots, onions, chick-peas, and so on. Pass through a vegetable shredder, shape, coat with flour, and grill with ground almonds, or cook *au gratin* in the oven.

Cereals are very economical as there is little or no waste involved. All the leftovers can be mixed, shredded, or minced for thickening soups or making *purées*. Any number of variations may be invented.

Sauces

Sauces to go with soufflés and cereal escalopes.

1. Fry an onion in oil. When the onion is golden, add water and a bay leaf, rosemary and salt, and cook (other spices may be used to taste). Then thicken with flour or arrowroot (yam root, sold by chemists or health food stores) and serve. If desired, the sauce may be puréed before thickening.

2. Fry chopped onions and raisins on a low flame. Use to flavour couscous or other cereals.

3. A cold sauce to replace mayonnaise. Eat in moderation. Goes with cereal croquettes. Cover malted or plain yeast with a little water. Leave standing for one hour. Add oil, salt, and spices, then whip.

4. The same sauce, but with the addition of soya flour. Cook on a low flame then add oil and spices. Serve with raw fruit or vegetables, and cereal.

Vegetable pâté

Vegetable *pâté* is a delicious alternative to any harmful delicatessen such as cooked meat. It is possible to be extremely creative and inventive with this dish, and it has the added advantage of being very economical. It can be made from cooked vegetable leftovers, or anything which might become stale, like lettuce or dandelion. These basic recipes can be modified according to season.

To make a good *pâté*, you need:

1. Good-quality bread which has been soaked in water, or flour. Vegetable oil. Spices, onions, shallots (optional).

2. Some vegetables: dandelion, pumpkin, leeks, carrots, mixed salad.

3. Dried vegetables: white haricot beans, azuki (red soya beans), lentils, kidney beans, chick peas, chestnuts (instead of flour) or mushrooms.

Mix the chosen ingredients in a bowl, pass them through the shredder, then place them in the oven. After cooking, add yeast.

Terrine of potted mushrooms

Place vegetable oil, onions, mushrooms, and toast or stale bread which has been soaked in water in a pan, and cook for 20 or 30 minutes. Add shallots, salt, and spices such as nutmeg to taste. Shred, then cook in the oven. While the mixture is cooling, add yeast (optional).

Dandelion pâté

The preparation is the same as above. Replace the mushrooms with dandelions and chick peas.

Vegetable sausage

This is accompanied by sauerkraut and potted *purée* of vegetables. Add buckwheat and lentils to vegetables and puree. Roll in breadcrumbs and fry. Chick peas, chestnuts, beans or flour may be used.

Dandelion or mash pie

1. Fry the dandelion in oil, then steam it. Carrots or onions may be added if required.
2. Prepare some pastry with flour, water, oil and salt. Cover a plate with the pastry, partly cook in the oven, then add:
dandelion and onions sprinkled with grated cheese. If the mixture is too thin, add shredded vegetables and thicken with arrowroot. Egg and/ or grated cheese may be added.

Pancakes

Add a little oil, powdered cinnamon or orange flower to the pancake mixture. Fill with apples, chestnuts or prunes.

This preparation, without cinnamon or orange flower, may be filled with mushrooms or vegetables. Having sprinkled the pancakes with a little grated cheese, place them in the oven.

One quarter buckwheat flour and three-quarters wheat flour may be blended with the pancake mixture. In the course of cooking the second side of buckwheat/wheat pancakes, sprinkle with grated cheese, fold over, and serve on a hot plate.

Clafouti

Prepare some stewed apples. Partly cook some prunes or dried apricots which have previously been soaked together with raisins. Mix the apple and the other fruit, together with the water in which it was soaking. Thicken with arrowroot, and sprinkle with ground almonds.

Couscous

Cook one cup of couscous in 2½ cups boiling water. Spice with cinnamon, orange flower, and a little vanilla. Blend with a little oil, and cook. Serve hot, with roasted almonds, stewed apple, jam, honey, or a moderate quantity of brown sugar.